Richmond upon Thames Libraries

Renew online at www.richmond.gov.uk/libraries

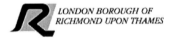

LONDON BOROUGH OF
RICHMOND UPON THAMES

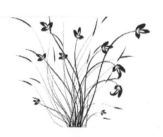

What people are saying about this book

"As an oncologist, I know that every time I tell someone they have cancer, I am starting them off on a unique journey. Although I can (and do) tell patients about all the possible side effects from their recommended treatment programme, I can never predict exactly how each individual person will experience these or which measures will be most helpful in supporting them through their treatment.

"That is why I am delighted to see this book in print. 'One Step at a Time' is a collection of useful hints and tips from the real cancer experts – the women and men who have been through treatment already. I hope that you will find it useful as you either set off on your own journey or support a loved one through theirs."

Dr Ellen Copson Bsc, MB BS, PhD, MRCP

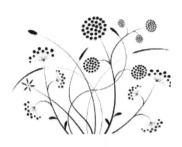

"Written by patients for patients, this book offers real insight of the 'roller coaster journey' that comes with a breast cancer diagnosis. Although an individual journey, these testimonies give honest and personal views on what you may experience, ranging from treatment, coping with emotions, advice, hints and tips. I hope reading others' experience will in some way help.

"In 2008, I was diagnosed with breast cancer. My journey has included surgery, chemotherapy, radiotherapy and various hormonal treatments, along with a number of setbacks.

"With the help of some of her patients, Alison has compiled this book to try to take away some of the unknown fears that come with a breast cancer diagnosis."

Lisa

"I think it's also a good book for family members (like me) of people having chemo to read too, as it does take away some of the fear of the treatment and makes you realise that it's not always as bad as people think. It leaves you feeling somewhat more in control than when you first started reading it."

Deborah

About the Author

Alison Bailey RGN
Breast Care Specialist Nurse at
King Edward VII's Hospital, London

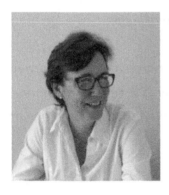

I was first drawn to working in oncology while I was a student nurse at St Thomas' Hospital in London. There I met a woman who had been diagnosed with breast cancer and showed such strength and fortitude in the face of her diagnosis, that it left a strong impression on me. Soon after that, in my early twenties, I travelled to Australia and worked on a haematology and oncology unit. I realised the long-term nursing care required in these instances opened the door to a type of nursing that I really enjoyed. I completed the oncology course at The Royal Marsden Hospital and started working with patients having chemotherapy. I have worked for 24 years in this area and have seen a huge change in the administering of chemotherapy, as well as the control of the side effects.

When a patient is diagnosed with breast cancer, it feels important to do whatever I can to mitigate the panic around the situation. I know I can't take the disease away, but I know that what I say and how I say it is an important part of how I care for my patients. The diagnosis can sometimes make patients re-prioritise their lives by wanting to be closer to family and friends, choosing a different career, or generally changing aspects of their lives which have been unfulfilling.

I strive to give them a realistic sense of hope and try to keep the focus on what they have control over at that moment, which is where the idea for the book came from. A patient said that, despite all the information that had been provided by the professionals and the internet, she would love to be able to dip in and out of a book that had useful advice for newly diagnosed patients, based on the experiences of other patients.

I decided to pursue this and canvassed the opinions of patients under my care, asking if they felt having such information available in this format would have been beneficial. The response was very positive and so I set about compiling and distributing a questionnaire to both NHS and private patients. I would like to stress that the information given is from each individual's personal experience. What works for one person may not work for another. Respondents have been wonderfully honest about the emotional impact of their diagnosis, treatment and what practical help is most useful.

It was pointed out to me that I have not mentioned breast cancer in men. This is because I simply have never looked after a man with breast cancer so had no way of collecting information. There are some patients who have used complementary medicines in conjunction with their prescribed treatments. I have provided the link at the end of the book to the Cancer Research website, which has information about complementary medicines. I would advise any patient interested in using these medicines to discuss it first with their oncologist.

The aim of this book is to provide a source of comfort and reassurance as well as practical advice for those given a diagnosis of breast cancer and their supporters (there is an extensive 'Glossary' at the back).

It has been encouraging having patients reading a rough draft of this book and telling me they wished they had it while they were going through their treatment. Knowing it could make a difference has kept me focused on completing it. My hope is it will become readily available for people with breast cancer going through chemotherapy, and that it will help patients and caregivers alike.

I have omitted names of patients, consultants and nurses, and as far as possible have quoted patients directly. I would like to thank all my colleagues at BMI Sarum Road Hospital in Winchester, the Royal Hampshire County Hospital in Winchester, the Spire Hospital in Southampton, King Edward VII's Hospital in London and Bridget Lubbock for their wonderful support with this project. I would also like to thank Dr Ellen Copson Bsc, MB BS, PhD, MRCP for her invaluable input, advice and encouragement. Many thanks also to Patricia Drew for the illustrations.

Most of all, I would like to thank everyone who filled in their questionnaires during or after an extremely traumatic passage of time in their lives. Their willingness to participate in order to help others was humbling and without their input, this would not have been possible.

Alison Bailey RGN

Dedication:
For Fergus, Rob and Gemma

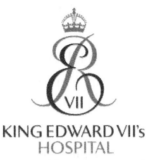

KING EDWARD VII's
HOSPITAL

This book is made possible in part thanks to King Edward VII's Hospital, who contributed to its publication.

King Edward VII's Hospital is a charity which opened in 1899 to care for wounded officers returning from the Second Boer War. Today, the hospital is committed to caring for all ranks of service personnel and their relatives, and to maintaining their reputation as the hospital of choice for anyone seeking the best private medical treatment in London.

The Breast Centre at King Edward VII's Hospital provides a full breast care service for anyone worried about their breast health or needing treatment for breast cancer. The centre brings together an expert team of specialist consultants, breast care nurses, and other clinical professionals to provide wrap-around care which meets all a patient's physical and emotional needs. This fully integrated service ensures that each patient receives the right assessment, diagnosis, and treatment as fast as possible.

Getting through Chemotherapy
for Breast Cancer

One Step
at a Time

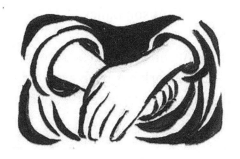

Written by patients
to help others learn
from their experiences

Compiled by
Alison Bailey RGN

Surrey, CR0 4PA, United Kingdom.
Telephone +44 (0)20 8688 2598
www.filamentpublishing.com

The right of Alison Bailey to be recognised as the author of this work has been asserted by her in accordance with the Designs and Copyright Act 1988.

ISBN 978-1-911425-01-4

Printed by IngramSpark.

This book is not intended as a substitute for the medical advice of physicians. The reader should regularly consult a physician in matters relating to his/her health and particularly with respect to any symptoms that may require diagnosis or medical attention.

Table of Contents

This comes in different forms, emotional and practical, from family and friends and organisations that specialise in this field. No single response is the same, but the underlying message is that support, in whatever form it takes, is essential.

Chapter 1 – Diagnosis

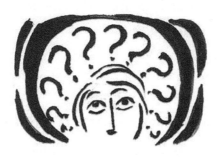

*T*he initial shock at being diagnosed with cancer cannot be underestimated. On many occasions, I have been a chaperone for consultants in clinic with patients who have just been told that the lump/pain/ sensation/discharge, is, in fact, malignant. I can only imagine what the words coming from the consultant must sound like. I have been told by patients that it is like a never-ending stream of bad news culminating in their worst fears realised.*

This chapter will aim to provide some comfort for new patients and show that there is plenty of support available in many different areas, there are no right or wrong reactions, and that the nurses and doctors are there to help in any way they can. One particular comment in this chapter that resonates is the quantity of unhelpful websites that are available and the need to obtain helpful information from the best possible sources, i.e. your surgeon and breast care nurse. I would also recommend all information required is taken from Macmillan, Breast Cancer Care and Cancer Research UK. The links to these are at the end of the book.

Diagnosis

"My first feelings were that of shock and disbelief, but even at that initial meeting, I did leave the hospital with assurance that surgery and treatment were available to help me make a full recovery."

"My initial diagnosis was made at my local hospital following an appointment to my doctor having discovered a lump. It was a breast clinic, there were a lot of people there and I was sent for various tests and then told to wait in a waiting room for the clinic nurse to call me in to discuss the results. I was very matter-of-factly told that the results were positive and that I would be given an appointment with the consultant a week later (the next clinic date) when I would be told what surgery/treatment I would need or be offered. The only good thing out of that horrible day was that it was so much part of a process and you felt you had been added to the conveyor belt, that having breast cancer was almost an everyday occurrence. That was all right until you left the hospital and had peace and time to absorb the information."

❧

"I was very glad that no one quoted five-year survival rates and statistics at me at any time. I do understand that some people may find it helpful, and perhaps in different circumstances I may have too, but for me and in my particular situation it wouldn't have helped me. I had expected it to be almost the first thing that was said to me and had been dreading it."

❧

"At my initial diagnosis, I was in complete and total shock so listened to what I was being told but only took in about half. Luckily my husband was with me so I asked him to go over what had been said later (in fact, I asked him time and time again until I remembered!). When the initial shock had started to clear, I researched as much as I could prior to each step of my journey. Being informed and in possession of the facts helped me to feel in charge and things that happened were less of a shock.

"Much of what I read was helpful but I always stopped reading if I found anything too worrying.

Forums were great – they gave me information from people who had been through the things I was going through."

❧

I would recommend taking someone with you to the appointments at the beginning. They can be an extra set of ears and take notes. The volume of information given and the shock of receiving the diagnosis can mean that most of what is said is forgotten.

❧

"Re diagnosis – I think the worst aspect was when hopes were raised, only to be dashed later. At my initial consultation with a GP, I was told that it was a harmless breast lump and that he'd eat his hat if it was cancer.

"The consultant then seemed to agree and told me that it should go away by itself. I was given an appointment for a check-up a few months later and told that it would probably have gone by then. I was further reassured by a clear mammogram. I hadn't realised that you could get false negative results.

"Then after the fine needle test results showed abnormal cells, cancer was rather starkly confirmed during an ultrasound. Obviously this was a greater shock than it might otherwise have been. I was then told it was very unlikely I would need chemo. Each volte-face made it harder to then accept subsequent reassurances."

Consultants and the need for information

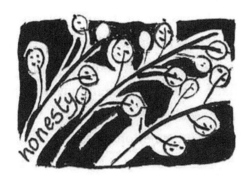

The consultants are there to answer all your questions, however insignificant at the time you may think they are. Some patients are eager to gain as much information as possible, which can bring a sense of security. Others would rather not know too much detail and leave the whole process to the doctors. There is no right or wrong way, just what would make you feel supported. Everyone takes comfort from fast treatment and clear communication, so do not be afraid to ask anything you are unclear about.

"The general feeling was that surgery and chemotherapy would work well with the size of the tumour; both my surgeon and oncologist were reassuring. The breast care nurse at my hospital was absolutely wonderful."

"The consultant surgeon assured us that he had removed the lump and it hadn't spread much further, so I felt that the cancer had 'gone' and that any treatment I was going to have was to prevent it coming back. I felt I was being given as much treatment as possible. The breast care nurse also gave me loads of information to read."

"The thing I do not like at all is uncertainty so the best outcome for me was confirmation of the diagnosis quickly. I see this 'illness' as a great opportunity to 're-arrange my life', to find out who I am and what is important to me and, as a result, be happier. I may therefore see things in a different light to other people."

"Only that the prognosis seemed to be good, given the nature of the tumour and that mastectomy was the best option, given its size. Clear and calm discussion."

"I have always felt it had been helpful to me to be given all the information and facts relevant to my cancer, to help understand what I am dealing with, such as my consultant oncologist giving me figures regarding percentages regarding full recovery with or without adjuvant treatments."

"Every person I came in contact with at my hospital was kind and caring. At the first appointment, my consultant said straight away that he thought it was cancer. So although waiting for further tests and results was the longest week of my life, it was not a complete shock when I had the final confirmation."

"My consultant saying eat what you want, when you want, as you don't want to permanently remind yourself you are unwell."

"My consultant saying ignore well-meaning friends and theories on what you need to do to get better."

This is a recurring theme throughout the book. Access the correct information from respected sites. All details at the end of the book.

"We are confident that we had good surgery, chemotherapy and radiotherapy were belt and braces."

❧

"I found the chemo nurses and my consultant extremely reassuring. What was new and frightening for me was familiar for them and they all excluded confidence that I would get through the process.

"That was really important. At the same time, the nurses were open and honest about the unpleasant symptoms I might experience. I found this reassuring also, particularly when the symptoms occurred, and rather than panicking, I could recognise what was happening to me from the descriptions."

❧

"The oncologist told me that the vast majority of people survive breast cancer which was very comforting and reassuring."

❧

"I think one of the most helpful things I was told at the outset of my chemo was when my consultant told me it was a year out to invest in my future. The other thing I would add is that life does go on – new patients should definitely realise that although the experience isn't one you would choose, you can still do things – go out with friends, take part in family life.

"Although I was careful, I certainly still did lots of the things I would normally do, everything from school concerts and parents evenings through to some part-time work.

"I personally think it is very important not to 'mope' about and feel sorry for yourself. Yes, it's horrible, and yes, I certainly did a lot of 'why me?' but you can't change it and you have to fight back and not let it completely take over your life."

"I was relieved and reassured by the informal and relaxed nature of my consultations with my consultant and the chemotherapy nurses. It somehow took the edge off, although I can't really explain what I mean anymore than that."

"I was very reassured by my consultant's openness during my first consultation. He said, '...and then you'll be fine' (I do understand that there are absolutely no guarantees). Of course, this is what everyone wants to hear, but knowing that doctors don't say anything lightly, I was enormously encouraged, and pleasantly surprised (delighted) that he actually did say it."

❧

"My specialists were able to answer questions about my treatment and side effects well."

❧

"The speed and kindness with which I was treated from the visit to my doctor, to see the consultant, to my operation, then onto the oncologist. I was treated with complete honesty and compassion and felt that everyone was on my side.

"As far as the surgical side, I found the help of the breast care nurses invaluable. They could answer all the questions that we were too shell-shocked to ask our surgeon at the time of the diagnosis and were available anytime I needed them if just to listen. I had a nasty wound infection, which delayed chemotherapy, so had a lot of contact with them."

❧

"Needless to say, we were profoundly shocked when first told that I had terminal cancer and no one could understand why this should have happened to a fit and healthy 63-year-old. When the consultant took over my case after some months, he was very honest and told us that treatment had to start immediately. I found his complete honesty and openness very helpful as I am not a person who wishes to be kept in the dark."

ഇ

"Better information about possible long-term side effects would be useful."

ഇ

"My condition was picked up at the breast screening unit after a routine mammogram.. I liked the doctor and her matter-of-fact attitude with me. I liked too that the core biopsy was carried out immediately with an appointment to see the surgeon made the following week. The doctor put the facts carefully, and initial comments regarding what would happen and the likely prognosis were absolutely accurate. She stressed the fact that so much was known about breast cancer that the oncoming treatments were likely to follow a pre-ordained course and that the outcome would hopefully be positive."

ഇ

"The comments 'one foot in front of the other' and 'this too will pass' and 'keep breathing' (Forrest Gump). A surgeon said: 'Lots of patients say "I just want it be over" – and then it is. Time will pass!' The surgeon also said cheerfully, 'I'll see you at the other side of chemo,' – confident that I would get through it OK."

"Meeting the surgeon, oncologist and nurses and knowing that they were going to be there to guide me through the whole process was a huge comfort and relief to both of us."

"My consultant's secretary mentioned that he was one of the best in Europe, and after some digging around on the web, that was confirmed."

"The initial pre-chemotherapy discussion with both my consultant and chemotherapy nurse was truthful, honest and therefore there were no surprises."

"My oncologist couldn't have done any more to prepare me for my chemotherapy and made himself very available to answer any questions I had without making me feel silly for asking."

"My GP said to treat the chemotherapy like a friend and to just take any possible side effects as merely a short-term inconvenience. Chemotherapy comes with such horror stories that one is led to believe that sickness and nausea are inevitable. This, I know, is not so.

"When I was first diagnosed, my consultant said to expect the worse and hope for the best and together we will deal with whatever we have to. Our family has adopted this as our motto for life in general."

The nurses

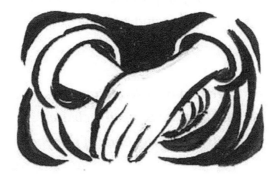

The nurses working in this speciality will provide their patients with all the information they need. Just occasionally, the information is not clear or not enough. I hope this section will give readers further material so they will have a better idea as to what questions they need to ask.

"With regards to meeting my chemotherapy nurse for the first time, I was put at rest by the fact that she knew how to put a needle painlessly in me and get blood out of my arm the first time round! That gave me confidence in her skills. Also the fact that my children were there and were not upset about it all means a lot to me."

❧

"Unfortunately there are so many websites that are either not helpful or do not relate to my cancer and therefore it has been so important to obtain honest and true information from the people treating me. It is also true to say that being reassured by these people is equally important, as you believe you are going to get better and life will return to normal again."

Take advice from nurses –
look at recognised websites.
Details are at the back of the book.

❧

"All the nursing staff were so comforting after both operations and throughout my treatment, and I needed that so badly. I remember looking at my breasts for the first time (after surgery) and just breaking down crying, but a lovely nurse sat with me for five minutes comforting me and reassuring me things would get better."

❧

"Knowing that I could contact the chemotherapy nurses or my consultant if I was concerned or worried about anything, however small. All advice was helpful."

❧

"Having a smiling face, a laugh and plenty of patience helped me to get through a difficult experience.

"Treatment at my hospital was fantastic, very approachable and helpful in all areas. Both chemotherapy nurses were attentive and caring and a well-run hospital made appointments flexible to tie in with my work hours."

❧

"The overall impression is of being on a roller coaster with relentless important information being given. Always take someone else with you to help remember what has been said – two brains are better than none! The information was given with great care and no question was too small or insignificant, every extra piece of bad news always had a good side, such as the fact the lymph nodes which had been removed were all clear, or the fact that the tumour was reactive to hormones so I could have further treatment.

"I was made to feel that however bad it was, there was always a positive side."

♀

"The word chemotherapy terrified me more than anything else. The vision of me as an archetypal cancer patient feeling so unwell with no hair just came to mind when I was told chemotherapy was necessary."

♋

"Chemotherapy nurses were very reassuring, exuded confidence and made me feel (rightly) that I was in very capable hands. They reminded me that they had seen many other patients who had got through chemotherapy. They provided lots of helpful hints and advice."

♋

"The oncology nurses were very helpful in advising side effects and helpful in advising low iron levels and what to eat."

♀

"At the time, it had not been determined as to whether or not I would be having chemotherapy, but we found it helpful to see where it would take place if it were prescribed and the nurse was very positive, emphasising the things I could do rather than things I shouldn't e.g. DO have a glass of wine if you want one; DO keep eating your normal diet; DO continue exercising normally while you feel like it etc."

❧

"Having the breast cancer nurse present was very reassuring. It was very helpful being given a contact number because after the initial diagnosis, your mind becomes blank. The Macmillan booklets are very useful."

❧

"They confirmed I was not alone and that they would guide me through all I needed to know. I felt information overload and was so worried about not timing something correctly or missing something. It was good to know there was a team of people who deal with this every day with hundreds of other people who were there to guide me through all the stages."

❧

"It must be very difficult to explain what might happen to a patient when one is dealing with the unknowns. Unfortunately because it is now the practice to explain everything very fully, the list of symptoms which are possible could become what one would focus on. If only the whole process can have a more positive press so as to make it less frightening. Chums who relate the horror stories of friend's bad reactions make it so difficult for those embarking on the process. I think it is essential to accentuate the positive i.e. the chemotherapy is part of the healing process which may cause short-term problems. It is almost as if someone suggests you look poorly, one could feel not too well immediately."

I cannot stress enough how important it is to ignore friends who recount horror stories about people they know who've had chemotherapy. There is nothing positive to be gained by listening and very little relevance as everyone is different. No two people have EXACTLY the same response.

"The nurses were amazing – so positive and friendly, you can tell they really care."

"All the staff at my hospital were very friendly. You become such a regular visitor, you see so many staff."

"My chemotherapy nurse for being able to find a vein so that I did not need to have a Hickmann line or Portacath 'installed'!" (see 'References' at the back of the book for the link to the Macmillan website which explains fully)

౭

"I was given some fact sheets which (necessarily) detail all the side effects you could possibly get. Reading these made me feel physically sick and once read, I didn't look at them again. In fact, I was given a selection of leaflets and booklets with loads of information which I found impossible to read in advance of treatment. I preferred to get information verbally from the oncologist and nurses rather than read it in black and white. This is not to say that the information isn't useful, but it was some time into treatment when I felt ready to read it. It's important to remind yourself that side effects are not compulsory and it is unlikely that you'll get all of them. In my experience, the anticipation was far worse than the reality."

౭

"Might be useful to be able to talk to people who have been through treatment. Fear of the unknown makes chemo seem more daunting."

The forums on the breast cancer charity websites can be helpful with this, or your chemo nurse may be able to ask another patient undergoing the same treatment to give you some advice.

"I would recommend your local Wessex Cancer Trust or Macmillan Centre to anyone. After walking in last week feeling so low and awful, I just poured my heart out to this lovely lady who had never met me before. She just listened and was so understanding. It is not the kind of thing I would normally do but I just had to offload that day and they were great."

"Nurses for reassurance and advice."

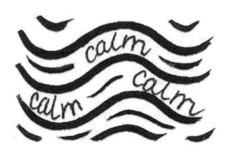

"Encouragement from nurses, their positivity and humour were infectious.

"My nurses' advice about not repointing the south-facing wall when I felt well has become a byword in our house. That is one of the hardest effects to cope with, coming to terms with the fact that any little thing takes it out of you and that you can't keep going at the same pace as always."

The nurse mentioned in the above comment was me! I stand by this statement; resist the temptation to do too much when you feel well, as it is not uncommon to then feel worse a day later.

"Nurses were good in a practical way and specialists helpful and informative."

"I think I could have done with a session with either a chemotherapy nurse or someone who had been through it before. The best help was speaking to a friend's friend who had just finished treatment. There are so many side effects that are hardly mentioned that it would have helped to know about."

"Some advanced tips on controlling side effects would definitely have been useful. Also more (clearer) information on what to do and what might happen if you become neutropenic and get sick (as I did) i.e. hospital isolation set-up, what and how monitoring will take place (chest X-rays, swabs, ECGs during temperature spikes), antibiotic administration etc. I found it a particularly scary experience as I had no idea what was going on or what to expect. For those with children, it might be worth encouraging them to make an emergency plan for such an event as we had to scramble to get it organised."

If you have not been offered this service, do make sure you ask the nurses at your hospital to put you in contact with a breast care nurse or a specialist chemotherapy nurse and ask them to explain what happens should you become neutropenic. They can also give you as much information as you want about the chemotherapy and what happens when you have treatment.

"For the whole three years, the nurses in the chemo unit have been wonderful. They treat you like a friend and do everything they can to make the whole experience as normal as possible, with no fuss.

"It becomes a part of your life. I feel so lucky to have such wonderful people caring for me."

"The hugs and chat from the nurses has done a lot to help me feel valued and cared for, especially now as my friends think I am all better so I try not to talk about it."

❧

"Nurses are a mine of information which I like. Also, a good laugh."

❧

"There's a fine line when you're feeling scared and vulnerable where on the one hand too much sympathy can make you feel even more scared, but on the other, a no-nonsense, practical attitude can seem uncaring. All the chemotherapy nurses I met, without exception, were able to tread that fine line with exceptional skill.

"They exuded a positive, friendly, professional, caring and reassuring aura which was totally calming and made me feel that I could relax and let them take care of everything. Amazing. Sympathy and practical advice being available on the end of the phone means you never have to feel that you're dealing with it alone."

❧

"All the staff I came into contact with were very kind, but they can't promise you everything is going to be alright, which is really all you would like to hear. I would have welcomed more information from fellow sufferers. I was given a copy of a book on breast reconstruction which was helpful but most of the views expressed by patients in this book are very positive and I would have liked with hindsight to hear more about the negative aspects of breast reconstruction.

"I think if I'd had the opportunity to talk to people who had had the surgery, I might not have opted for immediate reconstruction or not the reconstruction that I had. Perhaps more effort to put you in touch with information on the internet would have been helpful."

"Overall the bit I struggled with was the decision to have or not have chemotherapy. I found that a really difficult decision and one that I felt ill-equipped to make. Maybe one suggestion for people like me would be to talk to others that have been through it; I would be more than happy to talk to anyone. I have never had any regrets about that decision. I think the' what if' would have haunted me."

Your consultant can explain the risks and benefits of chemotherapy and can give you as much information as you need. It can help if you take a list of questions with you; they are there to help and will be only too happy to answer them.

༄

"I've only just found out that I'm entitled to free prescriptions. which would have been useful to know."

༄

"The breast care nurses were always there to help and arrange care, treatments and appointments."

༄

"Wonderful always, cheerful and complementary (when I felt otherwise)."

༄

"My initial meeting with my consultant was very informative and did not feel rushed. Both my husband and I walked away feeling that he had been honest with us. I have always found him to be very approachable and easy to talk too. Likewise the chemotherapy nurses reassured and helped me, especially important on my first chemo session, when I felt so frightened."

"I think exactly what was going to happen could have been explained more clearly. Things like how the chemotherapy was going to be administered, that I would be sitting in a room with other patients receiving chemo, how long it would take, that I would be offered coffee and could take in a laptop and log onto their internet. I turned up for the first session knowing none of the above."

"Everything I was told at the pre-chemo discussion was relevant and true and was explained in a sympathetic yet realistic way. The dangers of infection during the chemotherapy process was very strongly emphasised to me which I did find a bit frightening, but certainly focused my attention and meant that I took all the necessary (and probably some unnecessary) precautions to ensure that I didn't suffer any infections throughout my treatment period. I went home feeling a bit apprehensive but OK."

"Their (the nurses) experience, knowledge and smiles is the best resource book you will find for everything you need to know about your cancer... and other things for that matter! Ask them anything."

Chapter Two – Chemotherapy

*T*his chapter describes in detail how the treatment affected each person. Some of the women I have treated over the years have commented that they could not have survived treatment without working, mostly part-time. Others have said never in a million years could they have got through the treatment and worked. Everyone is different. These are opinions and information that might help when you start.

I would advise any patient starting chemotherapy to come with someone else the first time. Not only can it help with anxiety, it is better to let another person drive you home as no one knows exactly how the chemotherapy is going to affect you the first time.

First, we look at side effects common to most chemotherapy drugs, and then we will look at the effects specific to:

- FEC (Fluorouracil, Epirubicin, Cyclophosphamide)
- AC (Adriamycin and Cyclophosphamide)
- Docetaxel (Taxotere)
- Paclitaxel
- Radiotherapy

When did you start to feel unwell?

"I felt unwell the first night and the following day. This was mainly retching although I was not actually sick. The first dose of chemo made me very foggy and light-headed. Probably not a good idea to drive. Once I had accepted the pattern of treatment, it made it easier as I knew the symptoms were temporary. (Having the nurse on call at this time was a huge relief.) I also used a digital thermometer if I felt under the weather."

A raised temperature can be a sign of infection, one of the side effects of chemotherapy. It is generally advised to make sure you have a good functioning thermometer. Please refer to Macmillan Cancer Support for further information.

"Usually two to three days post-chemo, I felt very unwell and this usually lasted up to a maximum of nine days."

"For the first two treatments, I felt rather tired the first three days of the treatment and didn't really eat or drink much. This changed to a week after the third treatment, with me not drinking much at all so I had a headache as well as feeling nauseous."

"Sick and tired for several days after steroids and anti-emetics wore off."

"Two days; it went on for approx three days, then I gradually felt better."

"I felt fine throughout."

"First day tired, second day fine, third day tired."

"The third day of a week was always the worst and normally after a sleep and plenty of food and then the steroids, it got better as the week progressed."

It started...

"Usually straight after chemotherapy. Nausea would last two or three days. Tiredness could last a lot longer."

"I think the first dose of chemotherapy was the worst – I felt so tired and nauseous after it. This was partly because we didn't realise I could take both sets of anti-nausea tablets. I thought I could but my husband said otherwise; we should have clarified this with our chemotherapy nurses before we left after the first chemotherapy and they had offered to write down the doses. After that first time, the nausea was far more manageable."

"The second phase of chemotherapy was relatively better. Although, by the end of it, I found it hard to swallow the pills. The hot flushes were bad and used to happen a lot at night. I had a lot of mouth ulcers and my teeth gave me a lot of trouble. My ankles were always really sore on waking but got better throughout the day. This continued for a while and has now almost disappeared."

Feeling unwell...

"Started about three days and lasted five days. Tiredness lasted the whole time."

"Six to seven days start up to fourteen, week three usually OK."

"I had two different chemotherapy cocktails, each for four weeks. The first lot made me feel incredibly sick for four to five days after each treatment and I was extremely sick after the first treatment. Looking back, I think my body must have been in some kind of shock. I couldn't keep anything down, not even water. Even though that initial setback didn't reoccur as my consultant changed the anti-sickness medication, I can safely say that I spent the whole time feeling nauseous. Once I got onto the second cocktail, those symptoms abated to be replaced by problems with nails and some muscle pain, but that was much more bearable and not such a big issue. I continued to have mouth sores and digestive problems throughout all the chemotherapy. I absolutely hated the effects of the steroids which made me exhausted and hyper at the same time. I couldn't sleep whilst on steroids for four days around each treatment and gained weight unnaturally."

Weight gain, I've noticed, is a concern for some women in addition to the other side effects of the treatment. Once the steroids are stopped, most patients find the hunger pangs reduce and they have been able to take control of their weight and diet.

"I didn't feel particularly unwell during treatment apart from a few bouts of nausea, usually four to five days after the treatment and probably bought on by overdoing things. It is important to know your limitations, which perhaps I did not as I was pretty determined to carry on as if nothing was happening, hich, I have to say, I think is the best option.

"If you work, I would definitely recommend working throughout treatment, if at all possible. It keeps you in a routine and gives you a good reason to get up in the morning."

"It started pretty much the next day and lasted for about five days. I was not sick but felt very tired."

"During chemotherapy, my usual pattern was that a few hours after I would get a migraine-type headache and feel completely out of it. This would be a bit better the next day, but then I would have hot flushes and go orange (I was allergic!). I then seemed to have an energy boost where I would inevitably do too much followed by a crash and then by about the middle of the second week, I was coming back to normal. Each one of the course got a little bit worse than the last and other side effects got worse as each treatment went on."

※

"For me the side effects of the chemo were combined with the recovery of the operation. I have had a lot of pain and stiffness from the operation and at times the muscles seemed to go into spasm and stay rock hard for hours, or most of the day. I was having physiotherapy at the same time as the chemo which helped, but the immediate effect was often to make me more sore. I do think these feelings were worse when I was suffering the tiredness of chemo. Everything seemed to compound itself to make some days very difficult."

※

"With my second type of chemo, I felt worse. It would start a few days in, and some symptoms a week in – metallic mouth, burning mouth, sore nails and balls of feet. That would go on for a week. Not debilitating, and little or no nausea, just unpleasant and tired."

※

"I am probably lucky that I didn't generally feel unwell during my treatment. A bit tired on the day of treatment and maybe for a day or so afterwards but then I was OK. The two big areas that I struggled with were 'the hair thing' and my taste buds which were completely messed up and everything tasted of metal."

❧

"A little dizzy for the first two to three days."

❧

"It varied between my different chemotherapy treatments but always after the first three days. I put it down to the effect of the steroids. Then all the side effects kick in and last until about a day or so before the next chemotherapy."

❧

"I felt a bit nauseous the second day after treatment and started taking the anti-sickness tablets straight away before it took a hold. I did suffer from constipation for a day or two but my GP prescribed something to take the day before chemotherapy and the symptoms improved after the first two sessions. After a few days, I suffered loss of taste which initially lasted about a week but got worse as time went on and unfortunately I could not find anything that helped."

❧

"I was very lucky throughout my treatment and didn't suffer the sickness that often accompanies chemo. I would feel tired and 'off' for about a week after treatment but couldn't have said if anything would make me feel better. This would last for a few days."

✒

"My hair began to thin 14 days after the treatment and I came home from the chemotherapy very tired. For the first week, I drank plenty of liquids, otherwise my urine became very acidic and made me have a cystitis-like feeling and almost thrush. Drinking plenty helps to alleviate this."

✒

"The second week after treatment, I feel much better, not so tired and with more energy I have found that I have acidic saliva which develops after a few days and I use Vaseline on the corners of my mouth to counteract the soreness. A lifetime avid reader, I find I cannot concentrate on this currently. Wine is not as delicious as before, Cinzano Bianco tastes delicious; I found that I prefer sweet things."

✒

"During the first few days, I had GI symptoms, varying between constipation and diarrhoea. After the second week, I had sore hands and feet which continued throughout my treatment. I also had fatigue and exhaustion during the afternoons and evenings from early on in my treatment and had difficulty sleeping at night. At times, I had nausea and mouth ulcers."

֍

"The side effects developed into a
recognisable pattern."

֍

"I felt reasonably good for the first 48 hours, then disorientated and dizzy from about day three until the next week's treatment. Sometimes nauseous, some days were better than others."

֍

"As I can remember, the worst days were two to three days after treatment – but it only lasted for a couple of days – but towards the end of my treatment, I did feel worse."

֍

The cumulative effects of the chemo can exacerbate the side effects of the treatment as it continues. It has often been said to me that the fatigue towards the end can be overwhelming. My advice is to rest as much as you need to.

"For a couple of days after each treatment, I just felt a bit fuzzy and tired. Downhill from day three (nausea, heartburn) for a week after first treatment, but it went on for longer after each one. Final week was mostly OK though."

"Four hours after the treatment, I had nausea and sickness and was very tired. The nausea lasted for a couple more days. I had aching hips and limbs for three days after that and constipation. I felt tired and foggy for up to two weeks and then felt better during the third week."

"I have to say chemo was horrible but bearable. Just go to bed – when in a normal day are you allowed to do that? Treasure the time you are getting to rest, mend and rebuild."

FEC (Fluorouracil, Epirubicin, Cyclophosphamide) chemotherapy

"I'm a very lucky person as I did not get many side effects from the treatment (I was on Epirubicin and Cyclophosphamide)."

❧

"Session one and two of FEC, I felt unwell approximately five to six hours after treatment (very tired and sick) which continued for the next 48 hours. After that, I gradually felt better and back to normal after five days. A few mouth ulcers seemed to appear into the second week; after, the roof of my mouth became rough so I started using the mouthwash straight away."

❧

"After every dose of Epirubicin, I felt unwell almost instantly and was often hanging over a bucket on return from hospital, although I was not actually sick. Losing my hair was for me more traumatic than being bald. As my hair was falling out, the hair follicles were really tender which surprised me. The veins in my arm gradually got more and more tender and getting the needle in was the worst bit. Having had the chemotherapy via a Hickman line made treatment much more bearable."

"First time, first chemotherapy (the red one – can't remember the name) started a few hours in. Subsequently I discovered supplements and alternative therapies. Suddenly I didn't have any periods of feeling unwell, and I'd simply feel a bit tired. I'd go home and get on with things fast, before the crash happened, and I'd still be waiting for it to happen days later. Never did."

"With FEC, nausea began within one to three hours and lasted for four to five days. I found by days five to six, it was much better. Terrible taste with FEC too. Hair loss began on day 14."

"Very low/depressed about day 10 to 14 with FEC."

"On the day of treatment, day one, I felt OK but didn't feel confident enough to drive myself home (20 minutes away), just felt a bit disengaged. Had no nausea at all, able to eat a normal evening meal.

"Day two felt OK, but again not confident to drive myself to the health centre for injection. No nausea and able to eat normally.

"Day three, felt a bit spaced out, tired, disconnected. I felt as though I was doing everything in slow motion as though underwater, tired. Started indulging in afternoon naps. No nausea, mild heartburn. Able to eat normally.

"Days four to six largely the same as day three but gradually feeling more with it. Tired. Day seven onwards, I felt virtually back to normal and able to drive, go walking, shopping, etc."

(The "injection' is neulasta... a drug given to boost white cell counts. Full explanation is in the 'Glossary'. – Alison)

෨

"Fine for two days. Then ill for about five days."

෨

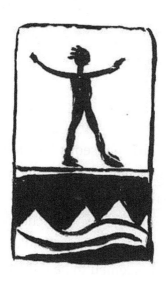

Adriamycin Cyclophosphamide (AC) chemotherapy

"The effects of the AC doses were different from the Paclitaxel. The AC chemo took 24 hours to kick in. The first night wasn't too bad but then the second night there was very little sleep but too tired to actually get up and do anything about it. The constant feeling of nausea is in the background, a cross between jet lag and morning sickness. The thought of food is awful but you know if you don't eat, you will feel worse. Meals cooked by friends at this stage were a great bonus. The effects slowly wear off, and after four or five days you start feeling a bit better, ready for the next dose. In amongst all this is the hair loss, which was not too bad, and my consultant's advice the day before the second dose was to have your hair cut as short as possible; certainly was useful."

❧

"The first chemotherapy (AC) I had on a Tuesday and I felt slightly nauseous for the next three days. By Saturday/Sunday, I became quite emotional (usually tears if I was left on my own to think about things too much). As the chemotherapy doses continued, my eyes watered and were irritated and my taste buds seemed to be dulled. Both these side effects finished after the end of the AC chemo."

❧

"Felt debilitating tiredness about three hours after treatment for a few hours, then queasy and tired for about five to six days. At its worst around day three. Lost appetite in general, but definitely went off sweet foods."

❧

Docetaxel (Taxotere) chemotherapy

"With the T (Taxotere), it was about three days after my first treatment that I started to feel the effects. I can't remember now how long I would ache for."

"Docetaxol much worse. Nausea much less on day one to two. Terrible aches and sharp pains began day four to five and lasted for about five days. Fatigue not too bad for me. Watery eyes plus on day 14. Still got. Eczema on face and hands days seven to eight to day 20 plus. Terrible mucositis with Doxetaxol day three to four to ten plus."

&

"Days five to ten, I felt low."

&

"On the day of treatment – day one – felt OK, but didn't feel confident enough to drive home. I didn't get the same feeling of disconnection with the world that I had after FEC. No nausea and able to eat normally, but felt tired.

"Day two – felt OK.

"Day three – muscle and joint pain started in the afternoon. Not really painful, just uncomfortable but it made sleeping difficult. I was advised that I could take paracetamol to relieve discomfort and aid sleep, which did work. Muscle and joint pain continued for three days.

"Day six – I thought I had oral thrush, but a visit to GP confirmed that it was 'white tongue' which made food taste a bit different and I was advised to brush teeth and tongue regularly throughout the day. Continued until end of chemotherapy treatment.

"Day seven – my hands started to itch and look red and swollen and quite sore. My face was also red and blotchy. I was prescribed Vitamin B6, which I took three times daily until the end of chemotherapy treatment. No side effects from these.

"Day eight – a mild case of diarrhoea. Days nine to ten – hands still sore.

"Day 11 to 17 – hands flaking and peeling like sunburn.

"After second cycle of Docetaxel, I suffered horrendous constipation on days three to four and any other symptoms paled into insignificance. My dose had been reduced so I didn't suffer the sore hands this time. Also at this point, my sense of taste started to disappear. It started with not being able to taste sweet things and then salt disappeared shortly afterwards. Foods began to taste metallic or had no taste whatsoever, and there was a metallic taste in my mouth all the time. My sense of smell didn't change.

"It was a very depressing time as, for someone who likes her food, I looked forward to meal times and now it was a struggle to find anything nice to eat. Fruit was OK as were vegetables, but all meat, cheese, fish, crisps, peanuts and puddings were hopeless. Lemon flavoured yoghurt was about the only sweet thing I could taste. This went on until about a week after my last cycle of Docetaxel, at which point it slowly started to return. Bliss!"

One morning I asked this patient if there was anything I could do for her. The response was, "If you see my taste buds lying around, could you give them back to me?"

"After third cycle of Docetaxel (same reduced dose), I suffered a recurrence of mild muscle and joint pain on days two and three and a red blotchy face on day four which lasted for four days. This wasn't as bad as last time, and plastering on plenty of moisturiser seemed to help."

৵

"Found this a bit worse but then it is cumulative. Fine for two days still and then ill for about seven days – slowly regain energy but never making it quite back to the starting point before having it again."

Paclitaxel chemotherapy

The side effects of Paclitaxel include nail problems. One possible way of avoiding these is to paint the nails with dark polish (preferably water-based, which has fewer chemicals in it) as this can protect the nails. I have seen patients with sore nails who haven't felt that it is an important side effect to tell me or their consultant. It is vital that any nail changes are reported to your consultant to avoid further complications, such as infection or the nails lifting off, though I have rarely seen that as most patients report the changes before it gets that advanced.

"The effects of the Paclitaxel, the day and night of the treatment, were not too bad – a bit tired! But the second night was much more disturbed and patchy sleep and then the next day would be a bit of a wash out. After that, steadily better until the next dose, although the tiredness is relentless. The nausea is much better (only there if you do too much), but on the bad day of the week it is much easier not to have to do any cooking. The tingling in the fingers and feet crept up on me and I didn't really notice until about week six or seven. Another problem I had with the Paclitaxel was that the lining of my nose was thinned and I would have nosebleeds regularly. These stopped within a few days of having finished."

"The Paclitaxel, which was every week, seemed easier to start with. Somehow it was easier to get into a routine which made the time go fast and I didn't have the ups and downs of emotions. However my feet started fizzing within about ten days and haven't stopped! After three sessions, my consultant reduced the dose but my feet didn't get better and my legs started to ache and I struggled to sleep so got more tired."

"Generally OK throughout, though definitely under par. Suffered with nerve tingling in fingers (from about week three) which is not unusual, but it was much much worse in my feet (toes and instep) which I wasn't expecting at all. I became quite clumsy and keep kicking and tripping over things which bruised my toenails quite badly. Some of my toenails have since fallen off. I had indentations in, and thickening of, my fingernails which has now grown out."

"The side effects of Paclitaxel has been progressive with no let up. After the eighth dose (now reduced), my consultant changed drug to another Taxane.

This was a bigger dose. I felt no nausea and the tiredness kicked in after three days. Ten days later and I still have a lot of trouble with my feet and legs. My mouth is constantly dry, my fingers are tingling slightly and my eyes are watering again."

Radiotherapy

"Radiotherapy – very little reaction at all apart from localised redness and mild tiredness. The five weeks went by very fast. Compared to the chemotherapy, it was a walk in the park for me."

"Radiotherapy – was a breeze after chemotherapy. Just kept smothering myself in E45 cream!"

Chapter 3 – List of side effects

This chapter provides a wide and varied stream of helpful tips that I hope will give reassurance as well as information.

Certain foods, complementary medicines, dietary supplements and massage can all help. Side effect we will look at are:

- *Nausea and vomiting*
- *Constipation*
- *Mouth ulcers/taste changes*
- *Hair loss/wigs*
- *Fatigue*
- *Skin problems*
- *Random Thoughts*

Nausea and vomiting

On occasions, I have treated patients who have felt nauseated on their way into the hospital for treatment. Anticipatory nausea is not uncommon and there are various ways in which to control this. Ensure the oncologist or breast care nurse is informed, and they will be able to help.

"I found the nausea to be very like morning sickness in that eating a dried biscuit helped me feel better."

❧

"I ate little bits of food more often and made recipes from a wonderful cookbook called *Healthy Eating During Chemotherapy* by Jose van Mil."

❧

"If nauseous, try to walk! Or sit straight up."

❧

"Lemonade, sugary food, and tea and biscuits."

❧

"Peppermint tea, travel wrist bands for nausea."

❧

"The anti-nausea tablets worked well. I found that, as with morning sickness, eating something e.g. plain biscuits, helped lessen nausea."

❧

"Eating little and often helped me, although I did put on weight. Regular short walks helped. Ginger ale and drinking lots of water also helped to quell the sickness."

❧

"I would highly recommend any patient to contact the Bristol Cancer Care/Penny Brohn Centre for dietary advice that is tailored to individual food preferences and eating habits. I included more ginger, mint and turmeric in my cooking as these helped my digestion. I usually enjoy a tipple which I gave up but found an excellent replacement in Dorset Ginger, which is non-alcoholic, but very flavoursome and aids digestion. Drinks like Schloer were also good for a treat instead of wine, and were palatable despite the drastic changes to my taste buds during chemo."

❧

"Cold fizzy drinks, rest and more rest."

❧

"Pineapple, green tea, walking and aromatherapy."

❧

"I found boiled sweets helped. I found flavoured fizzy water was good, although I can't face the stuff anymore."

❧

"When I felt nauseous, it was better to keep eating a little. I found things like yogurt, pots of rice pudding or pots of custard slipped down well."

"Jacobs Cream Crackers for nausea. Had to be Jacobs – wholewheat, organic or anything other than Jacobs didn't work for me. Strange but true. One bite would calm any nausea instantly. Still works now on choppy sea crossings! I carried a little clingfilmed packet of them around the whole time."

"Loads of ginger. Ginger ale/beer/preserved ginger and ginger root capsules.

"Taking ginger root, which can be bought in capsules, helped with nausea."

"I found eating a cooked meal at lunchtime and a light supper helped with the nausea."

"Eating little and often."

"Lighting a smelly candle strangely helped to prevent the nausea."

"I found drinking peppermint tea and chewing Airwaves menthol gum helped."

ॐ

"With FEC, lemon cordial, elderflower, pineapple, melon."

ॐ

"Bland, non-spicy foods, sweet foods."

ॐ

"Perhaps avoid favourite foods at chemo – I developed an aversion to some of them. Cold food was tastier than hot. Water can taste disgusting post-FEC. Stock up with squash, juice and smoothies."

ॐ

"Surprisingly, the foods that helped me were spicy ones – fajitas, chilli etc.! I also craved carbohydrates (toast, pasta, jacket potatoes etc.) so much so that several times friends had to go and get me a Burger King! But that really did help and kept my strength up. I consequently did put on some weight but decided I couldn't tackle everything and the advantages of these foods far outweighed the weight issue! Now that I have finished treatment, I have returned to the gym and have lost a stone! Together with my new hairstyle (now that I have my hair back!), I love my new image which has boosted my self-confidence and made me feel 'I'm back'!"

"Have what you fancy and when you fancy it. If it is a Big Mac, then on this occasion embrace it and don't feel guilty about it. My body told me what it didn't want. Went completely off milk and (sadly) wine! Fruit teas were good"

"Don't cook yourself – easier to eat then."

Constipation

I've heard many patients comment that constipation is one of the more unpleasant side effects and, by nature, embarrassing to discuss. The only possible addition I would add to this chapter is to start treatment (in whatever form) as soon as any symptoms arise, if they arise, and try to take a little exercise if you can.

"I invested in a juicer and followed recipes from *The Juice Master – Keeping it Simple* by Jason Vale. There were recipes for everything! Constipation was a big problem and the juices really helped along with Movicol."

"Drink loads of water!

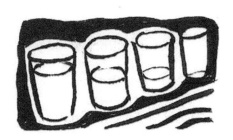

"To get rid of constipation, I drink a cup of black filter coffee first thing in the morning (plus it wakes me up too!)."

❧

"To take laxatives, as constipation was a problem after the first treatment."

❧

"I soon learnt to stave off the worst of the constipation by taking Senna tablets from day one of the treatment for two or three days, plus lots of fruit and water."

❧

"Laxatives (on day one and for two days after each treatment) and prune juice the rest of the time to stave off constipation and piles. (Was given

Magnesium Hydroxide Mixture by the hospital – this can be bought over the counter)."

"I found the best solution for me was glycerine suppositories."

"Movicol for constipation."

"Magnesium Hydroxide – stool softener for constipation."

"High fibre foods and loads of water – to help prevent constipation."

"Gentle exercise – I chose walking rather than going to a gym to help prevent constipation, to help keep energy levels up and for general well-being."

"Drink as much water as you can face, and I always had a Movicol the day before a treatment and then the day of and the day after"

"Tried various constipation meds but found the best thing in the end, apart from drinking plenty, was to move your body more! Get out of bed, walk as much as possible, or just do things around the house."

Mouth ulcers/Taste changes

Since chemotherapy attacks rapidly dividing cells, it can also affect the rapidly dividing cells lining the mouth, causing ulcers and taste changes.

"Taste buds were completely shot but I absolutely loved sparkling water with a slice of lime – very refreshing. I have attended therapies provided by Wessex Cancer Trust, which was much appreciated."

"I noticed that I could not drink tap water (as it tasted horrible), but that I tolerated sparkling mineral water the first week after chemo After that, I could drink my normal hot water (made with mineral water) again."

"My sense of taste has changed, and the first few days after treatment I have drunk low-calorie tonic water with lime, bitter lemon, or dry ginger, sharp but with a little sugar. It is surprising, alcohol is a no-no, and the very taste or a sip of red wine is disgusting, as is coffee at times."

"I could not taste spicy foods, such as curry or chilli, and preferred a slice of toast, soup or salad after treatment days."

"I found the taste issue really annoying. When you explain it to someone, it sounds so insignificant, but to be there day after day with a disgusting metal taste in your mouth is horrid. I had my teeth cleaned by the hygienist before I started treatment (recommended) and also use mouthwash every day, but I didn't find a way to make the taste go away. Eating spicy foods helped, but only in the short term.

"When the chemo affected my taste buds, especially at night, I sucked Starburst."

"Drinks with a fizz were the only ones that cut through the block in my taste. No foods tasted right and I discovered that I should stay away from spicy food as the spiciness seemed to be magnified.

Eating little and often also helps. Small, squares of Wensleydale cheese were good at taking away nasty taste."

"Lime cordial helped to remove the metallic taste."

"I used bongela inside my mouth if it was sore."

"Bonjela for the mouth ulcers. Embrace the taste changes – just have what you fancy."

"Avoid curries! I got terrible mouth ulcers which lasted for ages."

"I had mouth ulcers (particularly during the second half of treatment) and was unable to enjoy my food or drink. I found Corsadyl mouthwash effective for the mouth ulcers if I started soon enough."

"I did get ulcers in my mouth, and mouthwash from the doctor seemed to ease them."

"Aloe Vera toothpaste helped with mouth sensitivity."

"Chlorhexidine Gluconate Antiseptic Mouthwash was also recommended by the hospital and was better than the well-known brands as it is much less astringent. It is available over the counter."

✥

"Mouth ulcers: Eat soft non-acidic food and drinks through a straw. Mouthwash with soluble dispirin. Recently I found Oraldene mouthwash – it helps to dip a cotton bud into it and apply directly to all the ulcers; this saves you the taste on the tongue."

✥

"The only real problem I had was with mouth ulcers, which were most uncomfortable. Corsodyl mouthwash helped, but it is quite strong and can have a burning sensation. My dentist prescribed Difflam mouthwash which was very effective and much more pleasant to use."

✥

"Putting a Rinstead pastille in my mouth helped with mouth ulcers."

✥

"Manuka honey 25+ strength. I took it neat or with hot milk. It was brilliant for mouth sores and nausea, or just feeling tired."

"Found swishing Biotene moisturising mouthwash several times a day really good as it helped with dry mouth and prevented mouth sores."

Hair loss/Wigs

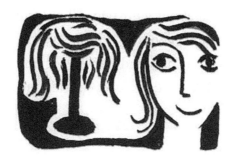

"Chemotherapy works by targeting all rapidly dividing cells in the body. Hair is the second fastest dividing cell and this is the reason why many chemotherapy drugs cause hair loss. The hair follicles in the growth phase are attacked, resulting in hair loss approximately two weeks after the commencement of the chemotherapy treatment." www.paxmanscalpcooling.com

"Wash hair properly before chemotherapy. Have the next wash two to three days after chemotherapy, avoid warm baths, swimming pools, and saunas for a few days after chemotherapy. Use lukewarm water when showering and avoid rubbing the scalp. Avoid

hot air when using a hair dryer, use gentle hair products and avoid brushing hair too hard". Scalp cooling: management option for chemotherapy induced alopecia, cited Auvinen et al (2010) Helen Roe. British Journal of Nursing, 11th September 2014

❧

"Be optimistic about your wig. All my friends could not believe how good it looked. Try on your wig at home so that a friend can see it and give you confidence. I did find losing eyelashes and eyebrows harder."

❧

"Don't think I'd try the head cooling again – but if it had been successful, obviously I might think differently. It just lengthened the whole process and made it far less pleasant."

❧

"Hair loss can be traumatic but more traumatic was loss of eyelashes and eyebrows. I never found a solution to that and tried false eyelashes and nearly blinded myself! There are 'Look Good Feel Better' workshops run by the Macmillan Trust."

❧

"Taking the 'hair thing' first, I know you all tell us that it will grow back and it does, but it is so horrible at the time and does take a while to grow back. I got very frustrated after my treatment that it wasn't growing back fast enough! My advice is to invest in a good-quality wig. Yes, when you first wear it you think everyone is looking at you and that you have a big sign over your head saying, 'Look at me,' but they're not, and you don't. For me, it was an absolute lifesaver. It meant I could go to the shops, talk to acquaintances, do normal things without anyone being any the wiser. You do have to cope with a lot of people telling you how fantastic your hair looks, but that's a small price to pay to have a normal life. I would advise seeing a wig specialist before starting your treatment.

"The other thing re hair is that I found using a coconut oil-based product helped my hair grow back strongly. Neal's Yard do a great hair treatment called Rosemary & Cedarwood which a friend bought me; this is coconut oil-based and very beneficial. The other thing is that if your scalp gets dry and flaky, washing it with Head & Shoulders works really well. My hairdresser was amazed at how well my hair has grown back. No strange texture or colour changes. She also commented that my scalp is very healthy with no problems."

❧

"Buff snoods or snood generally for heads!!"

❧

"A close girlfriend came with me to buy the wig. It was a horrible thing to do but she helped to make it fun and also made me choose the sensible wig, which when it came to wearing it was the right one. A girlfriend was easier than going with my partner."

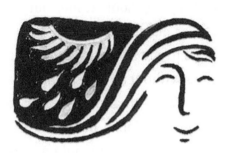

"I used a brow pencil to fill in missing eyelashes and eyebrows. Initially I used a dye kit from Boots which gave my brows more definition for longer."

"As much as you won't want to lose your hair, it is something that is best to address early. For me I knew that would be one of the worst parts of my treatment. Invest in a good wig, even if, like me, you buy it 'just in case' (I did need mine but always hoped I wouldn't). I had my bob-style haircut into a shorter, more manageable style for when I had surgery. I then went with my sister to an excellent wig shop locally where I tried several on in private with just my sister and shop owner who offered invaluable advice. I brought the wig home and put it away.

I wore it in front of some family members without telling them and because it was so similar to my new hairstyle, they didn't notice! Even when I told them, they were still doubtful until I removed it! I also wore it out for short periods initially, just to reassure myself that people weren't staring! When I started to lose my hair, it was there and ready. I think it would have been much harder to go out and choose one then when I was being 'forced' into it. I also chose to shave my head, which was hard, but my straggly hair by then looked so bad I would not let myself be seen with it anyway! Shaving my head made the wig much more comfortable too. I really would advise getting your hair cut short. That way, people get used to seeing you with your real hair short then don't notice when you progress to your wig.

Also, when your hair grows back (which it will!), it is much easier to then have it cut and styled in a short style ready to reveal rather than waiting for it to grow to the length of a longer wig or your original longer style.

I also invested in many (many!) hats. Ironically, I never usually wore hats as they ruined my styled hair! I found Baker Boy hats suited me rather than caps. I bought mine from Accessorize and eBay. They pulled down at the back and sides and you really couldn't see I was bald underneath! I did buy some false fringes which I attached to the front of the hats. I ended up with nearly as many hats as I have shoes! I am still wearing them even though I now have my own hair as they are perfect for the winter or the school run when you have a 'bad hair day'! (Yes, you have to get used to that again!)

I did buy scarves and bandanas but never wore them – they made me look ill! If you do chopse scarves, there is an excellent website called Annabandana which does them in so many colours, you can co-ordinate any outfit and they are very reasonable."

"The only thing I would recommend is that to get a wig before you need it as I found that the most devastating part of the whole treatment, although I knew it was going to happen. I did not realise how it would make me feel to lose my hair, and being able to put my wig on immediately helped. Also, if someone did suffer extreme sickness, they might not feel well enough to go and have one fitted."

"I didn't bother with a wig. I wore turbans and immediately had a grade one all over. It was so much easier and made the actual hair loss moment much easier. Eyebrows and eyelashes are gutting but they come back and it is only for a short period of time. All other hair loss was quite frankly convenient!!"

&

"The effect of losing your eyelashes, in my case, made my eyes and nose water uncontrollably, most disconcerting when in the middle of a conversation! The good news is that only a month after finishing treatment, I had a definite 'down' on my head and my eyelashes and eyebrows are growing back."

&

"My wig advisor told me about eyebrow tattooing, which has to be done before chemo starts owing to the use of needles and risk of infection, and often requires the consent of your oncologist. This is useful if you are worried about losing eyebrows."

&

"Before I started chemo, I was advised to go and get a wig, so that I had it when I needed it. In the end, I chose never to wear it but gathered a collection of headscarves and hats which were a mix and match and I chose to wear these instead. I found losing my eyelashes much more upsetting than my hair. I could disguise my lack of hair with a pretty scarf but there was no getting away from the 'cancer' image in the mirror. The 'Look Good Feel Better' programme (Macmillan) recommended eye pencils to draw eyebrows on and I also found using eyeliner on both the bottom and top eyelids helped add some expression around the eyes. You get a fab goodie bag from the workshop too."

Patients who went to these workshops loved them. It gave them a real boost and the added bonus was coming home with a free bag of goodies! The chemo nurses should be able to recommend a good wig specialist.

"I would have liked reassurance about being able to get suitable wigs etc. as I was really worried about this and losing my hair."

৵

"I was given the name of a good wigmaker, but what I was missing is how to look after my scalp now that my hair is gone!"

৵

"There wasn't much pre-discussion. Also, there was no info on wigs – a BIG thing for women about to lose their hair."

❧

"Go to the hairdresser or fit a wig if necessary. The local Macmillan centre can arrange home visits."

❧

"I never go out without my wig and make-up (tricks and tips provided by wonderful 'Look Good Feel Better' workshop). This all helps me to feel 'normal' on my good days. When indoors, I never wear my wig; there are some funny moments when someone knocks at the door and said wig is nowhere to be found!"

❧

"Hindsight is a wonderful thing, but looking back I would fit a portacath straight away and also cut my hair short before the first one."

Cold cap

"The cooling system works by reducing the temperature of the scalp by a few degrees immediately before, during and after the administration of chemotherapy. This in turn reduces the blood flow to the hair follicles, which may prevent or minimise the hair loss" – www. paxmanscalpcooling.com

There are differing views re the cold cap machine but the experience has changed with the development of new machines and better fitting caps. The cap is put on at room temperature and gradually gets colder, thereby avoiding the shock of the instant cold that was felt with the older models. It is hard for the first 10 to 15 minutes as the scalp cools down, then it goes numb. I feel able to confirm that, having experienced it myself.

"I chose to wear the cold cap during my chemotherapy sessions. You have to wear it for quite some time before the chemo is administered and for a while after too. I found the whole process really unpleasant but was determined to stick with it. Towards the end of the treatment, I did lose most of my hair but wasn't completely bald. I found that as I had some hair left albeit very thin and patchy, it did grow back fairly rapidly, so my conclusion on the cold cap was that it had done a reasonable job."

"The cold cap was not explained sufficiently – would have been nice to have known that the first ten minutes were the worst, and taking paracetamol will help. Difficult to read with the cap on, if you wear glasses."

"I remember my friend, who is a hairdresser, telling me to wash my hair in cold water 24 hours later to help close the follicles. It's also good to use a low chemical, neutral pH level shampoo." www. paxmanscalpcooling.com Website Patient Stories

Fatigue

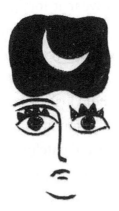

Based on the many patients that I have seen and treated, the side effect common to all of them is fatigue. The effects can sometimes be underestimated and I have seen how debilitating it can be. One of the quotes in this chapter is "surrender yourself to the tiredness" – a very good piece of advice!

"The worst side effect for me was the fatigue which continued through radiotherapy and took a long time to get over. I was fortunate and did not have too much nausea.

"Other less tangible effects are loss of concentration and memory (chemo brain) which can take some time to return and does make you think that you are going mad sometimes."

"I just carried on as usual but had a rest every day."

"Afternoon naps – brilliant."

"As yet, I haven't started the radiotherapy, but nothing changes in the way of tiredness! A friend has made a daily rota so that I will be driven to Southampton and back and so not have to worry about parking. I think that would have been a bigger stress than the actual treatment."

"I continued with yoga too, and found the mediation aspects useful when trying to sleep. There are cheap apps and free podcasts that can teach simple mediation techniques (headspace)."

"Surrender yourself to the tiredness but then get plenty of fresh air and exercise during the good days."

"Just go to bed. It's a treat."

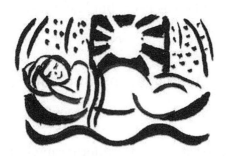

Skin problems

"Reflexology on my feet with lavender oil helped my feet plus Udderly Smooth foot cream. I used E45 on my hands at night and put cotton gloves on my hands to keep the cream on."

❧

"Loads of natural beauty products for skin.
Extra vitamins."

❧

"Reflexology at my local Macmillan Centre really
helped my symptoms."

❧

"For itching under the feet and hands, Piriton seemed
to help. I also put my feet in iced water.

❧

"My skin seemed very dry and baths with E45 helped a lot as well as being very relaxing."

❧

"With Docetaxol, Epaderm needed for my face and hands."

❧

"I used Palmers Oil for my scar. I used a lot of body lotion as my skin was very dry. I like the Dr Organics range from Holland & Barrett which is reasonably priced. The facial oil is great. The Body Shop also do some great stuff (as my friend said, they've come a long way from patoulli and bananas). I used a natural jelly, not vaseline (couple quid, internet), on the insides of my nose when it was sore."

❧

"For some relief from burning, throbbing hands after Docetaxel, fill (no more than two-thirds) a freezer bag with water and chill in the fridge. Put chilled bag in a container of suitable size to allow you to sit with your hands in, the bag lying across them. Not overfilling means the bag can mold to the shape of your hands more easily.

"To help with the healing of the above, I used the cream Eucerin recommended by the pharmacist.

Doesn't do anything for the pain, of course, but does really help to keep the skin hydrated and so prevent splitting. Longest lasting thing I have tried as it seems to penetrate the skin well."

❧

"I got really dry skin so have loads of moisturisers. Smother yourself in cream, particularly your hands and lips."

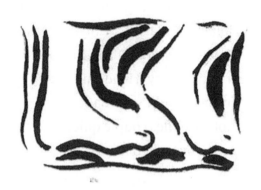

Chemo brain

"I would have appreciated if someone mentioned that as part of the chemotherapy, one's memory, ability to focus/concentrate could be affected and possibly give a suggestion that a notebook and pen ready to hand could be very useful. I don't know how much the chemotherapy has affected my memory, but it seems to be worse than normal and I do need to write things down a lot more. Luckily

I was warned about this by two Dutch friends who both had chemotherapy and still have issues with memory, focus and multitasking nearly six years after their chemotherapy finished."

❧

"I don't know whether it makes the treatment easier, but it certainly helps to anticipate the 'chemo brain' effects and be ready for it as much as possible.

A book that I can recommend is 'Your Brain after Chemo: A Practical Guide to Lifting the Fog and Getting Back Your Focus' by Dan Silverman and Idelle Davidson.

Random thoughts

I put this quote first as I feel that the internet can be as much of a hindrance as it is a help. As mentioned before, your consultant and breast care nurse are the best source of information, or recognised Breast Cancer sites if you need more.

"Keep away from the internet forums. It's very easy to scare yourself by reading other people's comments when you don't know their medical background, the regime they are on etc. which may make all the difference in the world to what they are experiencing compared to what you could reasonably expect. Generally there's a large proportion of depressed and depressing people who post on these forums."

⤚

"'Look Good Feel Getter' (Macmillan) free afternoon was brilliant and lifted my spirits. Free massages at my local Wessex Cancer Centre were also great."

⤚

"To get rid of my sore throat, I use herbal tea 'Throat Coat' (http://www.revital.co.uk/Trad_Med_Throat_Coat_Tea). I make a thermoflask (one litre) of this tea and sip it during the day until it's gone. I felt an improvement towards the first evening and did not need it after the third day (or I suck on Dutch liquorice 'muntendrop')."

⤚

"Sleep and going to work after the first week for the next two before the next hit."

⤚

"Keeping busy crucial!"

⤚

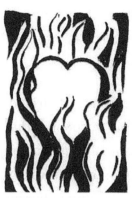

"Heartburn had been a problem so I have at times eaten smaller portions and not too late in the day."

"I have not tried any alternative medicines or dietary supplements but am going to start aromatherapy massage through my local Cancer Trust. I have never had any form of massage before but my neck shoulders and back to ache now."

"I have taken paracetamol and Ibuprofen when muscle pain had been bad and rely on half a sleeping tablet to help me to sleep at night, often because my head is full of thoughts relating to my experience with cancer. I have been concerned about the level of drugs going into me but know it is essential for me in the long run."

"Having a week away in between three months' treatment was a good feeling."

❧

"I was given LifeMel honey by a friend when I was first diagnosed and took a teaspoon of that every day from the start of my chemo through into my radiotherapy. Whether it really worked or I was extremely lucky, I never had to miss a treatment because of my bloods. I had Reiki healing and relaxation given to me on a regular basis, and learning how to meditate and concentrate on just your breathing helps to switch off the brain which often has too much going on in it to let you rest and relax properly."

❧

"Radiotherapy was much easier to deal with than chemo. No noticeable side effects from Herceptin."

❧

"Treats to look forward to like theatre trips / holidays are helpful. I took great pride in climbing Mount Snowdon two weeks after finishing radiotherapy, the month after stopping chemo."

❧

"Side effects for me were hair loss, nail loss (fortunately only on my feet), constipation."

"Acupuncture helped hugely to detox, and for general exhaustion and blood building."

"Reiki – hugely relaxing and healing."

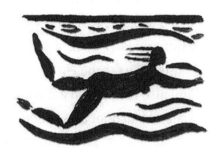

"Swimming in the sea, if you are able, made me feel revitalised and energised, and well and healthy and all things good. Like a normal person, not a chemotherapy patient at all. Supplements and foods daily that made me feel human included aloe vera juice, a shot glass morning and evening. All of these supplements made me feel as though I was doing more to help myself get better, and to counteract the negative effects of the chemo. They are also things I could continue after treatments had finished, and so gave me a feeling of empowerment over my own well-being. A massive thing, since I have subsequently discovered a lot of patients flounder once treatment has finished and they are discharged, since suddenly they are no longer 'fighting' their cancer and so feel vulnerable to it again."

❧

"What I would say is make sure you pamper yourself and eat a really healthy diet. I was bought organic face packs, creams etc. which were fantastic. I also ate (and still do) masses of organic fruit and veg. I really think this made a difference (I have a veg box delivered each week as this is by far the cheapest way of eating organic veg and also means you eat what's in season). I completely cut out alcohol and caffeine (apart from the occasional square of dark chocolate). In fact, a friend asked me what I was going to give up for Lent to which I said, 'I've got nothing bad left to give up!'"

❧

"I took a vitamin supplement and a probiotic drink each day which seemed like a good idea, but couldn't say if it really made any difference."

❧

"For shopping – always take a trolley to hold on to.
Back pain – hot water bottle.
Cystitis – drink plenty of cranberry juice and get a prescription for antibiotics asap.
I also took Vitamin C daily."

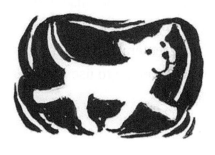

"Try to go for a walk, however short, every day."

❧

"A little of what you fancy (however fanciful!) does you good. Sleep and light exercise."

❧

"If I felt well enough, a walk in the fresh air or some gardening helped."

❧

"Aromatherapy at the local Cancer Trust Centre was very relaxing, especially on the day before chemo as I often felt very tense."

❧

"Shepherd's pie, homemade soups, lots of water, fresh air and walking. Eating out, swimming in the sea, shopping (taking your mind of the treatment), hand and nail cream."

"Hand sanitiser – I had my first session of chemotherapy delayed because I was fighting an infection (bad cold) and so became a bit paranoid about infections generally. Using hand sanitiser, and getting those around me to use it too, gave me some peace of mind."

"Never sit alone and scared – there's always someone out there to talk to."

"Don't be afraid to have a good cry if you want to. It's unrealistic to expect to be positive 24/7. The trick is to pick yourself up again afterwards and don't let it become a habit."

"Remember that thousands of women have gone through this, are going through this and will go through this, and you can too."

"Writing a diary. I left the left page blank to put in any good things that happened or were said to me. I could see them at a glance to cheer me."

"Without hesitation, I would have to say walking.
It made me stronger and kept me sane."

"I always tried to eat, even if it was a little bowl of pesto pasta. I use a lot of tea tree cream for various spots that appeared on my face and around my mouth. I used Bonjela inside my mouth if it was sore."

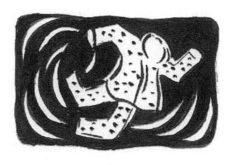

"I would advise ladies to invest in some decent pyjamas. Wearing them you can answer the door or sit in the garden for coffee with a friend looking presentable and not worrying about your skimpy nightie, but if you feel poorly you can hop straight into bed without needing to change! I had cotton button-down top-style PJs which looked like a shirt and trousers."

"My other side effect was weight gain. Not something I was expecting but again you just need to embrace it for the period of the chemotherapy and not worry about it. Far more important that you have a little of what you fancy when you want it to keep your strength up."

"Warm comfortable clothes when attending chemo, if you feel the cold, especially if you are using the cold cap, I would think".

"I always take a hot water bottle to every chemo as it works wonders with the veins, raises them up and I have no pain when the cannula goes in."

"Post-chemo, pack a 'just in case' emergency bag in case of admissions. Have a think about who would have your children in case of emergency admissions."

"From a practical point of view, it might be useful to mention to patients to see their dentist if possible before starting chemotherapy."

Chapter 4 – Support and help

What helped to get you through your treatment

*W*hen I see a new patient, one of the first questions I ask is about support – who is at home and does the patient need me to contact anyone for help. There is always a variety of answers. The first quote is a prime example of the need for healthcare professionals to be aware of the differing living circumstances of each patient. Some patients decide not to tell many about their diagnosis, mainly because they are struggling themselves and they don't want to hurt or upset their family or friends.*

I have been heartened by many tales of support given to patients from the most unexpected quarters and, it has to be said, disheartened by other stories of friends crossing the road to avoid any contact. The second example is not common but nonetheless extremely hurtful. It is important to realise though that this reaction usually occurs because people are terrified of saying the wrong thing. Generally the level of support I have witnessed by friends, family, work colleagues etc. has been unbelievable for the majority of patients.

It can be helpful to have a nominated spokesperson who your friends can contact for updates. This saves you having to repeat the same information to concerned friends which can become exhausting.

There are different forms of support mentioned in this chapter, and there are contact details for breast cancer charities in the reference section for further assistance.

- *Family and friends*
- *The importance of work and routine*
- *Think positive*
- *The professionals*
- *How my colleagues helped me*

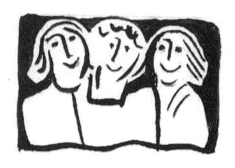

"This was more of a problem with radiotherapy but applied slightly to chemo too. I felt that not enough consideration was given to the fact that I live alone. (I was trying to say that when someone lives alone, there's no husband to call the hospital in the middle of the night when I felt terrible. And no one to pick up prescriptions, so it would be good if the medical team just assumed the worst and prescribed anything that might be required up front.)

"I would have preferred if doctors had assumed worse side effects and prescribed appropriately. i.e. heartburn drugs and loads of anti-emetics."

Everybody's circumstances are different and your sources of support may not be obvious. However once the sources are found, it is remarkable how much everyone wants to help.

ॐ

Family and Friends

Emotional

"My husband and children were definitely my inspiration for getting through each round of chemotherapy. I also decided not to tell everyone about my cancer. I kept it to a few very good friends and family. This way, I have not been treated any differently by those that don't know, which has helped enormously."

"Definitely the amazing family and friends I have; I couldn't have done it without their help. Everyone was so supportive; taking care of the kids, getting me to hospital and just generally being positive. The nurses were part of this too – seeing the same nurses every week certainly helped as you build up a relationship with them."

"Support from family and friends. Staying positive! If I felt well enough doing something special i.e. visiting family and friends, going for a meal. Leading a near normal life as possible.

"Support from a wonderful team of family, friends, the local Wessex Cancer Trust Centre, work colleagues and previous patients."

❧

"Support of my husband and wanting to be around for my two young children."

❧

"My mother was my rock and virtually moved in for the whole treatment. My daughters and my fiancé gave me the strength and reason to continue."

❧

"My family – it is they who could do with counselling and support for their fears. They carry a heavy burden and may feel their support goes unnoticed by professionals."

❧

"I think realising how many true friends I had who were prepared to put themselves out for me gave me a huge boost."

❧

"My daughter and my husband always being supportive and encouraging. Knowing that it was coming to an end. Honestly, I have found the recovery more difficult psychologically and emotionally than the treatment, and that is where I think perhaps more preparation is needed."

❧

"The support and friendship of those around me has really helped and has touched me enormously. My own mother was diagnosed with breast cancer at my age. She is now 22 years post-cancer and gives me great hope for the future."

❧

"What helped me through was definitely the support I received from my husband. It was fantastic, and also having my son around to show me that life goes on and we still have to deal with all the day-to-day things. I also read Prof. Jane Plant's book *Your Life in Your Hands.* I'm not sure if the medical profession see it as a bit controversial, but I certainly found it very supportive.

"Reading about other women who have experienced what I went through, and are still around 15 years later to tell the tale, makes you realise that you can get through it and come out the other side. I would definitely recommend it."

"My husband's unwavering belief, encouragement and support (even when bald!) and having my wonderful children around. When your children appear at your bedside in the morning wanting breakfast, you have to deal with it, no matter how you feel, and it is hard but it also takes the focus off of you and that, for me, was a helpful thing."

"My husband had had cancer and had a positive attitude."

"The emotional support from family and friends, plus the support given by the Macmillan Centre, where you can talk about things you can't always talk to your family about."

"Practical support is needed but it's the emotional support that gets you through."

Having friends to support me.
Being able to talk to someone.

"Without a doubt, the support of my husband. It was important that he was familiar with the chemotherapy routine as it was then that I felt quite vulnerable. I have a little saying which keeps me positive, 'If the mind believes it, the body will achieve it'."

❧

"For me, the thing that has helped me the most through this is the breast cancer care forum. By joining an online thread with people going through the same chemotherapy at the same time was invaluable. I have made some great friends on here. It would have been much more difficult to manage without."

❧

"My husband has been absolutely amazing! I know it's been difficult for him too, but he's always maintained a positive attitude – my young children have also been fantastic. My family don't live locally but have been as supportive as they can."

❧

"What has amazed me is how supportive and incredible my friends have been. I'm very bad at asking for help, so they just liaised with my hubby and ignored me!"

❧

"My children give me hugs when I'm down
and were pretty much themselves."

❧

"My friends and family have been absolutely
fantastic. It has been so important to me to talk
about my illness openly and I made the decision
to let everyone know at an early stage, so they did
not feel they could not approach me about it.

"My daughter's reaction surprised and upset
me but I understand now it has been her coping
strategy. She was 14 years old and had almost
belittled my condition, insisting as few people as
possible knew at the school that she attended and
I worked, as she did not want anybody asking her
about me. At times she blanked me and walked
away when I have tried to talk to her about it. My
son was helpful when possible, but admitted he
did not know what to say."

❧

"Everyone was amazing and so supportive.
Family, friends and partner give constant
care and reassurance."

❧

"Support from friends and family was a wonderful and invaluable help, although sometimes I felt it was me that was supporting them by keeping strong and putting on a brave face. I suppose they were in shock too. Bizarrely, as I am an emotional person, I rarely cried. I suppose I thought it would send a negative message. I had a great friend who went through almost exactly the same things two years before. She was the best support ever and I never felt I had to put on an act with her, plus she now looks amazing so I could see the light at the end of the tunnel. My friendship with a fellow cancer patient helped, comparing notes with our various experiences and hopefully this was a mutual help."

"Husband unfailingly positive, occupational health, GP – very supportive. Breast care nurses and chemotherapy nurses were also very supportive."

"I was very fortunate to be overwhelmed by emotional and practical support from neighbours, friends, work colleagues, my immediate family and all the medical staff I came across. I've never been so well supported in my life and I know that I've only got through this so well psychologically because my courage was constantly held up by others' helping hands. I wouldn't have got through without all this kindness – it reinforced my already strong belief in human nature."

∽

"Emotional and practical support from my husband and twin sister (who works at St Thomas' Hospital)."

∽

"Support from family and friends is paramount and maybe a suggestion would be more support for them. Certainly one of the most helpful things for me was going to the 'walk talk' group every other week. Talking about very personal things with others who have been there and laughing with them has been my greatest tonic.

"I wish I started going earlier and I would strongly recommend it. I went to counselling once, but found I was just talking about cancer. With the group whilst you talk about cancer, it is mixed in with talking about family, work, politics etc. and feels so much more normal."

∽

"My partner has been fantastic. He comes to every appointment, which is very important. To start with, I was in so much shock, I wasn't absorbing half that I was being told. Later as the journey became more emotional, he offered great moral support. His patience on days when I haven't felt so good, especially at night, has been unfailing – I could not have got through this without him."

❧

"My husband has been and continues to be a great support. It is not easy for the people around you that care, and one should bear in mind that you are not in this alone and it is very hard for people that love you as they feel powerless and helpless.

When, on two occasions, my hair started to fall out, he has shaved my head (emotionally stressful for him). He takes care of my medication, does the heavy chores in the house like hoovering etc. and makes sure I rest when needed."

❧

"My children are grown up and show me great love, as do my grandchildren and all family and friends. I consider myself very fortunate."

❧

"My friends at work and home were very supportive keeping in contact by email, text, telephone and visiting. They provided me with the emotional support I needed as unfortunately my husband initially was so upset, he seemed to be focusing on his own feelings instead of mine, which I found very upsetting. It was due to my friends and other family that I was able to stay positive and cheerful. Luckily he managed to conquer this in time to help support me through the chemotherapy and radiotherapy, and we celebrated our Ruby wedding anniversary."

"My family were brilliant – they didn't fuss over me but were just there if I needed them. Friends were brilliant as well and just popped in for a chat, but I knew they would be happy to give any help they could. They offered lifts, but I was well enough to drive myself. It was good to know help was on hand if required."

"My friends and family have been brilliant and it would have been difficult without them. I also met with a lady who had chemotherapy and that was the most useful."

"I receive a lot of help with childcare from my husband and family so that on the days when I felt tired, I was able to take it easy and have naps. My husband and parents quickly learnt that it wasn't a good idea to leave me on my own as I would dwell on things and normally end up sobbing."

"My sister was diagnosed with bowel cancer in 2010 and talking with her about her experience and emotions while going through chemotherapy (albeit a different combination of drugs) was invaluable. I said I was scared and she was able to convince me that none of it was agony (she didn't have the constipation I did!), just a hard slog. My husband was able to act as a really useful barrier between me and people I didn't want to see!

"VERY important: friends saying that they would be there through the whole process. I worried that I would get forgotten. Parents who took the time to explain to their children what had happened to me so they could help my children cope too. I knew that took courage and I was very grateful. School knowing my situation too.

"Writing emails to avoid too much exhausting chat. Having an opportunity to chat to a patient who had just finished her treatment and who was still standing! Hearing from the oncologist how the statistics showed that all the treatment made a big difference to my survival.

"All this information came from the computer and made me realise I benefited from tens of thousands of other patients' experiences, the realisation that I felt very loved and just how fantastic friends can be. A friend bought a chemotherapy cookbook, and there were lots of imaginative ideas.

"My friendships have deepened and lots of people have confided in me with their past experiences to help me. I have made some good friends too – it is very special when a friend you do not know too well helps you. The realisation that I was so much stronger than I thought; I have a lot more confidence in myself. Some time by myself to get my head round the diagnosis and to have a cry, but also knowing I would see someone the next day... plan ahead!"

❧

"Try to go out a little so that friends can see you and know that they can approach you. It made me happy after the school run just to have a brief chat, hello and a smile, and often people can only do this if you look them in the eye. In my case, this extra effort on my part paid dividends. I'd got out to school early in the treatment and then when I had my wig – it is another hurdle over and relaxed me."

❧

"Let friends know if you welcome plenty of texts or if you would like peace. In my case, it really helped me to know that people were thinking of me often."

❧

"Make yourself the most important thing – prioritise, look after yourself and protect yourself. Choose friends you see carefully in the early days. Use your instinct to choose positive and practical personalities.

❧

Try to spread the emotional load so that your partner is not too exhausted. Ask a friend to tell people; it is exhausting repeating yourself.

"What I enjoyed most so far is actually having the time to TALK to people, instead of running around like the proverbial chicken, and I get to know more people and acquaintances/friends."

"Being able to have someone to discuss my feelings, and feel I am not fighting the cancer on my own, has been very important to me. I find my fears and thoughts are stronger at night when I go to bed, so I have often needed to talk to my husband then.

"He has always been very supportive. I particularly remember when he clipped my hair for me, which was so personal and upsetting to me, but he made me go out that afternoon to a local shopping centre with my headscarf on to try and build confidence. I was glad he made me do that as it did help me to deal with the way I looked without thinking about it too much. I have a friend in Jersey who has just finished her adjuvant treatments for breast cancer and it has been good to talk and compare her feelings and experiences of this illness."

"When I was at my lowest, they boosted me taking me out to lunch, or just a chat."

"Having family or friend with you when you were having your chemotherapy treatment made the time pass quicker and my partner gave fantastic support throughout the two years."

❧

"Emotional support and practical help. Most helpful aspect, knowing that I wasn't going through it alone and relieving some of the worry about how to cope with looking after the kids during treatment."

❧

"Learn to accept help whenever offered. I found people wanted to feel as though they were doing something to help. I had a rota to drive me to radiotherapy, although I am sure I could have driven myself. The company was brilliant and I used to enjoy looking in the diary to see whose turn it was. In fact, my friends got quite competitive and the days filled up instantly. A team of girlfriends came and blitzed the garden, which was wonderful. I had regular visitors who came in for chats."

❧

"Short visits are good, great people wanting to come around to help, but I didn't want anyone except my close family for too long. Anything that people can do to help is great but it is also really important to stay in control. I found that if people tried to take over completely, that made me feel useless and really down. It is about a balance and people taking the lead from you. When I felt better, I wanted to do a bit more, not to be told to sit down all the time. Equally there were other times when I was left to do everything and I could not cope.

"Friends keep in touch via e-mail. It is a good way of keeping in touch, particularly on days when you don't feel like talking."

"I couldn't have got through it without my husband. He is always there, no demands or expectations but prepared to sit and listen when my emotions have gone out of control. Always ready to give me a hug and reassure me. Just having someone to say your darkest dreads to relieves the tension."

"Chatting to friends when forced to (!), not forcing me to do anything (other than chat), and NEVER deciding they knew best and forcing me to do something 'for my own good'.

"My husband accompanied me to almost all my appointments and chemotherapy sessions. It was helpful from a travelling point of view, but mostly for emotional support and as an extra pair of ears as I found it hard to take anything in and remember to ask important questions."

♋

"Tolerance and understanding to the fact that you can lose your confidence. Avoid telling me that I will be alright ... don't worry."

♋

"Overwhelming support from friends and family. Lots of visits from friends to keep my spirits up."

☙

"I did manage to keep the home ticking over myself but occasionally did not feel like driving or shopping so needed help with that, although online shopping was a godsend. Mostly, it was emotional support I really appreciated. Just to have a laugh with friends made all the difference; no one wants to visit a miserable person.

"My friends are always on the phone and are there when needed. A lot of local chums have offered to help with lifts to radiotherapy. I am trying to follow my own adage of asking for help from those who have offered it. I have also deferred from doing other things regularly, saying that I prefer not to commit myself at the moment."

"Sometimes I just needed someone to agree with me and acknowledge that it was traumatic and horrible! It's a natural thing for people to say and I don't blame them. I'm sure I would have said the same."

"Making sure I walked every day and chats with cups of tea (or a large glass of wine). Looking after the children whilst I was at hospital, and protecting my children. I was very adamant that my children should be aware of the treatment that I was going through but I wanted the facts to come from me, and not casual comments from other people. As I learnt myself, every cancer patient is different."

Practical

"Being able to carry on as normal. Working."

෨

"Having treatment at work – not having to take much time off "– has financial implications being self-employed. Having support from Macmillan unit, including therapies and 'Look Good Feel Better' service".

෨

"I was very lucky and received support from family and friends. They helped take care of the children, especially during treatment days and in the summer holidays when my treatment started. They also remained positive, which helped me. The school where I work brought some normality.

"My mother came over from the Netherlands as soon as she could after the first operation and stayed with me until after the second operation, and my brother stayed with me during both operations. We spoke about the operations and why breast cancer happens on a daily basis and what it can mean to me and how it can help me change my life for the better."

෨

"My husband came daily to the hospital and talked about his work so I had a link to the outside world and afterwards drove me everywhere until the time I could drive again. He came home on time to take the kids off my hands."

❧

"Friends helped looking after the children, texting me and asking how I am, offers of picking things up from Ikea/town etc."

❧

"Family and friends for shopping, driving me around, being there to talk."

❧

"Lifts to treatment both chemotherapy and radiotherapy. Meals cooked, children looked after."

❧

"Husband accompanied me for chemotherapy sessions. Friends gave my children lifts to school when I was most tired. Visits from friends. All invaluable."

❧

"Thinking back about help I received when I was ill, whilst I really hungered for contact with friends, often it wasn't as beneficial as it might have been

– some friends sent cards and gifts which was wonderful, particularly books, and one friend decided that chocolate was an important weapon against chemotherapy and would send regular treats. Less sensitive friends/relatives would ring and not take hints that I was tired, or worse still, descend unannounced and expect me to cater for them rather than offering to help with meals/drinks."

"Friends helped me with the practicalities. One had my dog for several weeks so I didn't have to worry about walking her. Another friend took over looking after my elderly parents. Every week they do their shopping and anything that needs fixing in the house like changing light bulbs etc."

'We had a lot of occasional help from family and friends with the children in the form of outings and play dates. This was great for them and a break for me/us".

"Telephone calls/emails and cards. I didn't want to know about any negative cases. My family and friends were great and work were understanding."

"Various family members stayed for two or three days after each session to help look after the children and produce meals. I lost my appetite so it was difficult to think about food, let alone cook it and eat it."

❧

"Overwhelming support from everyone. Friends visited, neighbours dropped by, the telephone was always ringing. Too much sometimes. Talking openly seemed to make me feel more positive. Offers of help with transport were always there."

❧

"Support included phone calls, visits, cooked food, flowers etc."

❧

"My husband has done a lot to reassure me how much he still loves me despite the change in my appearance.

"My friends' support was brilliant; they cooked for me, picked the kids up from school, went shopping and kept me busy. My sister was excellent as she had been through the same thing. The nurses were very good when I was in having treatment but

I would have liked a phone call on the first night from them to see if all was OK.

I had no inkling that anything was amiss before the mammogram result and so friends were shocked, as I was, but sympathetic, of course. Everyone knew someone who had been through it and I was bombarded with positive stories of recovery, flowers and good luck cards, all of which were helpful in the initial stages while we were coming to terms with it."

❧

"Email good friends your chemo dates so that they know when might be good to help/contact you. I am not normally good at asking for help but knew that I must so that my children and husband had a better experience. It helped me to accept all the offers."

❧

"Just after my surgery (bilateral mastectomy), lots of my friends cooked meals for my family which was so, so helpful. Friends have been round and taken me out for lunch or just popped in for a cuppa. My husband took on the house and childcare whilst I was having my 'bad days' after chemo. Having three children also keeps me going and is a great distraction from what you are going through. Friends also rallied round to help with lifts to and from school. People want to help, so you do need to ask and/or accept all offers."

❧

"Friends drove me to and from hospital for treatment while others looked after the kids and picked them up from school, meaning I could just concentrate on me and go to sleep when I got back from hospital."

❧

"My husband drove me everywhere for nine weeks after the operation after which I could drive again. He still takes me to chemotherapy (I just don't fancy driving home afterwards)."

❧

"My mother-in-law came down on a Wednesday afternoon and helped me with getting the kids to swimming, changed and getting dressed again."

❧

"My mother comes over every time for a few days around the day that I have chemotherapy to support me and talk about lots of things and helps cleaning the house."

"Friends have offered support from shaving the remaining hairs off my head (although my kids helped by cutting it shorter) to driving my daughter to Stagecoach (theatre art school) to taking me for a coffee and a chat."

"Most helpful was shopping and driving me to appointments. Friends and work colleagues visiting and talking about other things than cancer and treatment."

"My husband has had to give me a lot more practical support through this. Previously, I have always maintained the garden and house on a weekly basis. However, because of the surgery and treatment, there are jobs such as grass cutting and hoovering that he has now taken on. I could not drive for six weeks after the first surgery so was reliant on him to drive me around, although I have found myself walking a lot more which also makes me feel better. I do walk the dog now, but not the early morning walk as I find it very hard to get out of bed most mornings!"

"Friends who wrote to me or took me to lunch."

"Someone to cook, bring me books, do the shopping, bring flowers, send cards, talk and not avoid me."

"It's great to have someone with you on the day of treatment so that you can just put your feet up and not have to think about all the usual household chores. I had various people fighting over who was going to take the dog out – he has never been so fit! My brother made the helpful suggestion that I should treat myself for every bout of treatment that I had so that I had something to look forward to afterwards. I took this very seriously, although it did get rather out of hand towards the end when I finished up with a holiday in Italy."

"Just being there, unobtrusively. Doing house things, cooking, letting me crash when I wanted or needed to, and letting me be on my own."

"Help with the children was vital when I felt rough. It was also better not to bring them to appointments as far as possible as we found that my little boy (two to three years old) did become anxious about what was happening."

"Short visits preferable to long ones. Bringing a meal saves me the bother. Short phone calls, long ones are very tiring. Good supply of books always very acceptable. Help with driving especially over long distances."

"Help with cooking. Being there to talk. Sending me flowers cheered me up. Texts of support on the days I had treatment. Was given loads of scarves – not particularly helpful for hair loss but very handy now! I have a magnificent collection."

"Ongoing contact and help with practicalities – shopping, dogs, children etc."

"Having meals cooked was an enormous help. My husband loved cooking so I was very fortunate as I never lost my appetite – just didn't want to prepare it. I also had help with the housework and gardening which stopped me worrying about it."

"Taking me to chemotherapy.

"Just being there.

"Cooking some meals.

"Regular cards to say not forgotten; 18 weeks is a long time."

❧

"Lifts to appointments were most useful and occasional shopping. Oh and someone blitzed my garden a couple of times – although I could've done with more gardening help."

❧

"Cooking as you don't feel like it at all the first week of chemotherapy. Talking to family. Friends driving me to hospital. Family there at my treatments. Family and friends looking after my children and getting a gardener and cleaner in to help at home. Friends taking me out to lunch and shopping."

❧

"My friends have been hugely supportive, particularly in my quest to remain active. I am not a self motivator so the friends made sure there was always someone to walk with. I walked miles; this kept me fit and cleared my head. Like a lot of people, my family live far away; this made the friendships even more valuable. My mother-in-law has lived through a breast cancer diagnosis and was invaluable for support during my hospital appointments."

౭

"As a mum, my greatest priority was my boys. I didn't want my treatment to affect them anymore than it had to. I tried to keep routines as normal as possible. Although they obviously saw me when I was poorly, we tried not to let them see me at my worst as this may have worried them. We arranged for them to be collected from school by grandparents on days we knew I would be poorly e.g. on a chemo day.

I did a huge shop and stocked up on all the foods I knew they liked! I set up a box for each of them with the drinks and snacks they each liked for their school snack bag and put up a list of what they each ate for packed lunches inside the cupboard door so that other people could make their lunches if necessary. Many people said, 'Let me know if there's anything I can do to help,' (as they do!). I decided to take people up on this and enlist their help. I allocated jobs to everyone: my mother-in-law used to collect the school uniform on Friday night and wash/iron it and put it back in the wardrobe ready for Monday; a friend did my ironing on Saturdays; another friend checked the boys' school website and reminded Daddy/grandparents of upcoming events e.g. sports day; another friend checked my emails daily and deleted obvious junk ones so that when I logged on, I did not have hundreds to sift through; my sister supported the boys with homework and music practice."

"They kept things consistent and merry. Cancer was discussed but not workshopped or analysed. It was a topic but not an agenda item leader. I understood it was important to talk about it, but at the same time it was good to have some normal banter with those you love most. I used my time sat on the chemotherapy drip to spend time with friends who would accompany me, which made a bit of an event of it. I felt like I was gaining time that I would not have otherwise had with these friends because I would have been at work. It gave my cloud a silver lining."

"Different people did different things. I spoke about the cancer with girlfriends who had been through the same process and with my husband. That was key for me – to be able to be open. Two neighbours volunteered to walk my dogs regularly and that took the pressure off me. I still walked her but didn't feel obliged to go out for longer than I felt able. If I needed a lift, then I knew friends and neighbours would help and I set up a lift system with friends and neighbours to cope with the 33 trips to Southampton for radiotherapy.

"One neighbour cooked a meal for my family and that gesture was very kind. Many, many people sent cards and flowers throughout my treatment and these constantly lifted my spirits. My two sons often took the mickey out of me, and that also helped by making me laugh, and my daughter was very caring and loving. Most of all, though, I was very lucky that my husband was so incredibly supportive throughout, so I never felt alone in the process."

"My two boys (aged seven and ten at the time), and family and friends, were ultimately what got me through. I am still in awe at how they have coped with everything and were able to give me strength and support at such a young age. Make the most of your 'good days'. On my three-weekly chemo cycle, I found I was dreadful for one week, reasonable for the second week and good on the third week! I used to arrange to go out to lunch, pop in to see work colleagues etc. on my 'good weeks'! I used to spend all morning getting ready – deciding what to wear, checking there was no 'evidence' of my illness (e.g. adjusting my wig, making sure outfits covered up the results of surgery etc.).

"After I had been out, I used to come home exhausted, but was always proud that I had tried to carry on as normal! The numerous compliments from friends made me feel great – I was determined not to look like a patient!

"Being open and honest with people is essential, I believe. As a teacher, I was worried what parents would think when I suddenly went on long-term sick leave. I made the decision to ask the headteacher to put a mention in the school newsletter. Following that, I received many messages and cards of support, and knew I had made the right decision.

"Being honest with my two boys was crucial. We told them I was ill the same evening we found out ourselves. It was the hardest conversation I have ever had, but somehow I found the strength from somewhere and was proud of myself! We did use the word 'cancer' which initially shocked and devastated them. But then we talked them through and really tried to be positive. We kept them at home the following day in case they suddenly became upset or thought of questions they wanted to ask so that we could deal with these and answer them immediately.

"We then contacted the school and made sure that all staff involved with the boys were made fully aware of the situation. We dealt with one thing at a time with the boys – surgery, then chemotherapy, then radiotherapy. They did ask many questions, which we answered as honestly as we could.

"They were so supportive and just seeing them smile or giving me a hug really gave me strength. I managed to work my chemotherapy sessions around special events as far as I could by looking ahead and moving treatment forward or back a day if I needed to. That way, I still made sports days, concerts etc. on my 'good days'. This was really important to me."

"Family, friends and nurses have been fantastic but some people are better than others. My chemotherapy nurses' comment of not to listen to everyone else's stories was a very good piece of advice. Some of the throwaway lines have been interesting! 'You must carry on being completely normal!' I thought I was. It is good to try and keep busy, but choose activities that are not too demanding. A lot of knitting and needlecraft has certainly helped me."

"I turned into a bit of a hermit. There was so much talking about the cancer during hospital visits etc. that I didn't feel like revisiting it with friends, although in retrospect I wish I had because the few times it was forced on me, I felt much better after getting over the initial reluctance to chat about it."

"Support. An interesting point. I certainly received this from my husband (who attended all my treatments with me), but regarding friends, colleagues and family, my advice is to be selfish and only tell those people who you know you will get support from. I had a few fantastic close friends who visited, took me out to lunch/dinner, bought me nice things and were generally great. I did tell one friend who couldn't cope with it all and although I see her again now, I didn't see her at all during my treatment. In those cases, I would say don't waste your energies trying to make them feel 'better'. As one of my supportive close friends told me, 'You are the most important thing at the moment so you can't feel guilty or bad about how other people are when you tell them you have cancer.'

"Regarding other people that I didn't want to tell, well I didn't and they still don't know. Some people treat you differently when they know you've had cancer and I didn't want to be 'so-and-so who had cancer/is ill', I just wanted to be the person I've always been and be treated in the same way."

"The untold support that I received from family and friends, nurses etc. cannot be underestimated. Family support had obviously had the most effect. Although my daughters both live in London and have young families of their own, they made the utmost effort to come and see me and to try and include me in anything that would interest me. The support from my husband cannot be underestimated in what must have been the most trying for him. It cannot be easy watching someone whom you love going through chemotherapy and knowing there is nothing you can do to help. His practical help, taking over almost all of the household tasks, washing, ironing, shopping etc. was just wonderful, especially on the days when I just felt wretched, but there was nothing that he could do except be there. Also of great comfort were the emails, cards, and letters that I received, some from people that I hadn't heard from for years, all saying positive things and most importantly, that they were thinking of me constantly. I know without doubt, that all this has helped me through."

෨

"My friends have been great. Occasionally one gets a call and can tell immediately that this is someone who had built themselves up to making the call and who is desperately frightened by everything. You then end up trying to cheer them up; it can be very tiring. My husband has also found it difficult to deal with this type of call.

"It was dreadful having to tell the children. My daughter gave birth to our first grandchild the day before the diagnosis. Again, some people think that was dreadful timing but to the contrary, we found it the most wonderful diversion and rather put my problems into perspective. Telling my daughter of the situation just days after the birth was hard and we were very worried about her, although I had been staying and managed to have a quick word with her visiting midwife, whereas telling my son who lives overseas was unbearable. I cannot stress how supportive my husband has been and how much my situation is due to him. I do not think enough care is taken of the carer in this situation."

ॐ

"Huge support from all, and ongoing through what seemed interminable treatment."

ॐ

"Very good support initially (lifts, shopping) but offers have tailed off. I'm sure they'd help if I asked but I don't like to."

ॐ

"Family are distant. My sister has stayed a couple of times but I don't really like people in my house for too long."

ॐ

"I had a friend who was going through the same thing and talking to her helped. Someone doing the cooking and shopping was really nice. Endless texts and answer machine messages were not helpful. In fact, my sister got everyone to phone her in the end and she passed on the latest news."

ॐ

"My husband's unfailing sense of humour and support in listening to me talk about my symptoms was one of the most important things to me during this time. He was concerned and yet didn't suffocate me with constant enquiries as to how I was feeling. I was able to convince him that I was fine on my own, and his going to work as normal and not tiptoeing round me really helped to make me feel that I could cope.

"Girlfriends helped me by driving me to appointments, listening to me talk about my symptoms and sympathising about hair loss, eyelash loss and cosmetic problems, which my husband found more difficult to empathise with.

"Another really helpful form of support was that my friends completely understood and didn't take it personally when I didn't want to see anyone – either because I looked rough, felt tired, or didn't want to risk infection.

"They understood that I didn't necessarily want to go to confined public places like the cinema, crowded pubs and restaurants, and they didn't just turn up on the doorstep, they checked first either with me or my husband if I wanted visitors.

"Frequent text messages were welcome and meant I didn't feel abandoned while everyone else got on with their lives.

"As an aside, I found the most unhelpful and overused phrase from friends and family during the time of hair loss was a cheery, 'Never mind, it'll grow back!' While true, being told this every day didn't seem to comfort me while I was losing it."

"Try not to get too upset by other's reactions and emotions; unfortunately not everyone is able to cope with your diagnosis. For me, a person ignoring my diagnosis and not talking to me about it when this is my life was one of the most upsetting things. However, in general, people's kindness and support shines through. Having children who needed looking after definitely kept things pretty normal for me. We found it best to be honest with the children. The unknown is often scarier and their imagination can run away with them.

"I was never alone on my journey. My husband continues to be my rock and together with my children, they have all been my greatest support network.

"Although not possible every day, I am sure that, for me, keeping positive means that I am well and about to celebrate five years since my diagnosis."

"Taking everything a step at a time and trying not to feel guilty about not doing anything. Not having to worry about feeding the family. Having support from one or two good friends who bought me creams for hair loss etc. – something that I would be too embarrassed to ask for in the chemist. Having someone help with wig choice. Feeling that you weren't fighting it on your own!"

"The biggest challenge for me, as I am used to being so self sufficient, was to learn to accept my limitations and to take help whenever offered from others."

The importance of work and routine

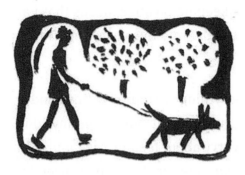

"Acceptance of the situation and knowing that I will come out stronger at the other end. I'm also 'working' with the treatment – I rest every day between one and three, I try to get as much exercise as possible, eat as healthily as I can (and feel like), spend more time with friends and family, and try to find out what makes me happy in this life."

ॐ

"Keeping on working."

ॐ

"Going to work and having the support of my colleagues whilst there made the year easier."

ॐ

"Definitely being able to carry on working helped a lot, and I was very fortunate in that my employers allowed me to adapt my working day to fit in with how I was feeling. You have to live your life as fully as you can, and not let it be dominated by the fact that you have cancer."

❧

"Having to wait for tests to see if there is any cancer left is absolute hell. The only way I got through all this was by putting it in my diary so I could count down the weeks. That is why, for me, routine was so important."

❧

"Without hesitation I would have to say walking. It made me stronger and kept me sane."

❧

"Calm and hugely unruffled. Being there without fuss and interference seems the best approach to me."

❧

"Maintaining a normal life. Continuing to work was hard but I was supported by everyone at the hospital and encouraged to work but to rest when possible.

❧

A smile and a hug helped me to keep going! Also having somewhere to go and talk was helpful."

Think positive!

"My cancer and chemotherapy journey has been very scary and your body goes through such an ordeal, but having a positive attitude really helped me to get through. However, I have also acknowledged my bad days and have had a big meltdown where I just didn't want to do chemo anymore, but actually felt better for it later, so you mustn't deny your feelings and accept each day as it comes."

"I believe a positive attitude and looking forward to the return of normal life has helped me get through so far. I have given myself goals to aim for to help me get through what seems like an eternity to me, one of them being to join a golf club in April and start playing regularly."

"We are all going down to Devon at half-term to give us a break, as although this is my illness, it has affected the rest of my family's lives as well. It also gives some normality and a defiance that I will not let cancer take over everything in my life. I have kept up with events at work and am focusing on returning as soon as possible.

"At the same time I have realised that health-wise I have to take each day as it comes, and if I feel unwell I give in and rest.

"As my daughter reminds me, it could be a lot worse!"

&

"My positive nature and will to enjoy life."

&

"Being positive about the outcome and getting on with normal life throughout the treatment."

&

"Whether side effect or actual menopause, the flushes and night sweats are constant from a few days after my first treatment, and if you have a sense of humour it helps because the side effects of even the Tamoxifen are... guess what, tiredness, hot flushes and night sweats... so what's new?! I have also been taking Menopace which is a multivitamin, but with all these things who knows what it would have been like without."

&

"Having finished my chemo and had three weeks off, I can't say I am looking forward to continuing with the Herceptin, but all these little hurdles are there to be scrambled over."

"Keep a positive attitude."

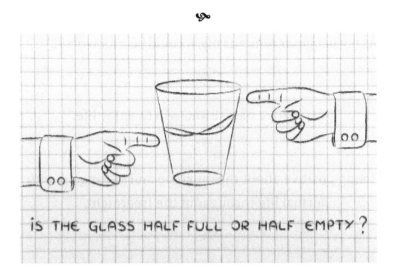

IS THE GLASS HALF FULL OR HALF EMPTY?

"Being a glass half-full person helps. It is much easier to be practical and cope with what is going on than thinking too much about 'Why me?!' My family and friends have been fantastic, always being there when needed, whether to make you laugh at yourself (always a good thing) or just around for a cup of tea and chat; there is nothing like it."

"Believing it was my best option and counting off the treatments. Meeting other patients and talking to them helped. It also gave me hope. I always wore my best clothes and made efforts with my make-up and perfume, manicure etc. I believe that if you look good, you'll feel good."

৽

"It has been a life-changing experience. I think it has made me appreciate so many things that I took for granted before, and much stronger to go out and get what I want. Cancer brings out the best and worst in people. You find out who your true friends are and they are not always the ones you thought."

৽

"Family, supplements, a new puppy (made it a very happy and funny year, rather than a miserable and scary one), and most of all, MOST MOST MOST of all, a positive attitude and a belief that this was not the end of me."

৽

"Trying to be happy and finding things to laugh about daily. Watching mindless comedy on TV, and lots of alternative therapies that detoxed and relaxed me, got the good hormones going in my system, and they made me feel positive, relaxed, happy and en route to healing. A lot to be said for happy hormones!"

৽

"Decide that life is precious. Take on new challenges. For me, I am learning to play the guitar and dancing the Argentina Tango. (The Tango was not easy and I had to push myself to keep going, but it has been worthwhile)."

"I remember our consultant telling us we needed to have things to look forward to see us through and how true that was. We bought a new puppy and the little chap kept me going; it made me get moving as he had to be attended to. We are also keen caravaners so we replaced our caravan and looked forward to the new caravanning season. I am also determined to see my grandchildren grow up. Something I did find helpful when I went for radiotherapy was contact with other breast cancer patients, and with hindsight I wish I had gone to the local support group run by the breast care nurses."

"Positive mental attitude is an absolute must! I am also determined that I am not going to be beaten by this beast inside me. I have too much to live for. My four grandsons are a great joy and I want to be here for as long a possible so that I can enjoy them growing up. Even though I have now finished treatment, I know that my friends and family are still thinking of me and their support continues."

"I always knew that life was for the grabbing and feel this more now."

"My GP told me to walk tall and keep my head up and that a physical attitude was as important as a mental one. Keeping your chin up is very important. I think that over the years, chemo has gained a bad reputation. I think it's time to change that; no more hushed tones when the word cancer is used. It is in so many cases merely a condition which the modern doctor in the twenty-first century has an arsenal of weapons to treat."

"I think what helped me through my treatment was being open about what was happening and talking about it, but also keeping other interests and not staying home alone feeling sorry for myself. I think it really helped me to keep doing things. I also made much more effort than normal with my appearance and experimented with different types of funky scarves tied round my head and still put mascara on my one or two remaining eyelashes!"

❧

"I think I personally felt the need to still look fine, so people wouldn't feel sorry for me and would still treat me like me! We also kept up our social life whenever possible, still entertained etc. So I guess, again, still keeping life as normal as possible. If I tried hard enough, I could forget it was happening!"

❧

"Having milestones to work towards. I counted down and celebrated each treatment being completed."

❧

"That third week before next treatment was enough to remind me what normal felt like and that kept me going."

❧

"Everyone wants you to stay positive and full of good humour throughout the process and it can be very tiring to put on a happy face 24/7. Support is helpful, but sometimes the 'stay positive, you'll be fine' messages can sometimes wear a bit thin when there are no guarantees."

❧

"Organise a coffee/walk with a friend most days; always have a little something to look forward to.

Try to be open so your friends can help you. It is difficult for them too."

"Just remaining as positive as possible helped me to be strong."

"Everyone is very understanding and I am trying to tell people that chemotherapy is not always as ghastly as people say. I think it is important to spread this particular word so as not to frighten anyone who may have to go through it themselves. The radiotherapy is pretty labour-intensive and therefore time-consuming."

The Professionals

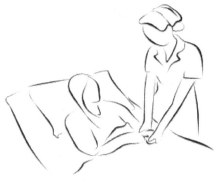

"When treatment is over, my chemotherapy nurse warned me that it could take up to a year to get back to normal. That was really helpful. I have friends that have had chemo etc. and expect to feel fine almost as soon as treatment stops and when I tell them it took me several months, they are reassured and stop pushing themselves so hard!"

"The chemotherapy staff, without exception, have all been incredible and just so cheerful, which has such a positive impact when you are going through chemotherapy. They make what can be a terrifying ordeal, so manageable, you almost look forward to chemotherapy sessions! Everyone I have come into contact with professionally have been honest, caring, factual and professional. No question has been too silly or stupid to ask."

"Friendly, relaxed and comfortable room for treatment. The care I received from the chemotherapy nurses in making sure I was comfortable and had everything I needed during treatment."

"Expertise of nurses – particularly my chemotherapy nurses' amazing ability to cope with my awful veins."

"My chemotherapy nurse did an amazing job of preparing me and then guiding me through my treatments. She was incredibly skilled and made the whole wretched business far more bearable. Every patient will respond slightly differently to chemotherapy and the insight she had gained from treating so many patients was extremely helpful."

"Incidentals. Chemo brain can take up to two years to go. I was advised by my chemotherapy nurse not to go back to work for up to six months, which was absolutely correct."

"Without any doubt, other people's kindnesses, thoughtfulness, openness and constant support – and total confidence in the medical attention that I received from everyone involved."

"The consultant's confidence that they were giving me the best treatment. At the end of the day, for me it isn't just the chemotherapy. I had surgery from which I am still recovering. My back, under my arm and chest are still very tight trying to get used to different muscles being in different places. The chemotherapy is there to kill off anything surgery missed. Towards the end of my programme of chemotherapy, the doubts started to increase about whether or not it had been successful and whether or not it will come back. Stopping chemotherapy is like having your stabilisers taken off your bike. You want to go to two wheels like all of your friends, but at the same time you are scared you will fall off your bike."

"Support from family and friends. Having days out and a holiday booked to look forward to. Walking every day. Magnificent, kind, sympathetic, helpful staff at the hospital where I was treated."

"My husband, of course, but without question it was the chemotherapy nurses. There was nothing I couldn't tell them and nothing they hadn't seen or heard hundreds of times before. Whether on the end of the phone or in person, they were always able to reassure me that everything I was going through, either physical or emotional, was completely normal and that many other women felt the same. I never dreaded turning up for treatment, there's always a happy, busy, fun atmosphere."

"Most helpful has been the Macmillan unit. They have made me feel that I can drop in at any time for support. Also support at my chemotherapy unit. Having lifts from people, most of all having company and meals cooked by friends. Just knowing that there is someone to talk to, particularly as I live alone."

"There is quite a large discussion on the side effects of chemotherapy, and this can leave you feeling rather depressed. There is a lot of information available on diet and life style. Whilst I appreciate that there are no clinical trials (yet), I thinking advice on diet and exercise should be given at the same time as discussing side effects, or guide people to reputable sources of information such as Penny Brohn or Macmillan websites. Also, there are some wonderful mastectomy websites, which have been started by inspirational people.

"Women need to know they can still look good in clothes. I still use some of my old bras with the fuller cup, and sports bras are good, and probably cheaper than mastectomy ones. If I have a low neckline, I just wear a vest underneath."

How my colleagues helped me

"My work colleagues from the start continued to email, phone and visit me, which meant I did not felt isolated and my boss had confirmed to me on more than one occasion that my position was safe."

"My manager at work is fantastic and she encouraged/encourages me to stay at home until the end of treatment so I can get properly better, and sent numerous cards, flowers and e-mails."

"Work colleagues' offers of help if needed – visits."

"Support from friends, family and colleagues was invaluable, although sometimes a bit overwhelming! One of the positive things about having breast cancer is that you do discover how nice people can be."

❧

"My work boss – paying for time off."

❧

"Colleagues were great whilst I was receiving treatment but when I reached the end, support evaporated very quickly as I looked well."

❧

"Work colleagues have looked after me too. I continued to work until the day of the operation. Since then, they have allowed me to work when I feel like it. I can do really mundane tasks to help generally in the office or do parts of my own job with no pressure. The ability to keep in touch with work without the pressure has been helpful and sometimes it is a lot better to be thinking of work than sitting around thinking about breast cancer."

❧

"Lots of offers of help but I haven't taken up many as I don't know them that well."

❧

"The best support they gave me was flexibility to work when I wanted. It meant I could keep going with work through the chemotherapy period which helped me keep life consistent, kept me having to look smart and think about things other than being at home or cancer, and ultimately kept my confidence intact."

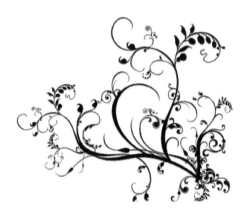

Appreciation of the book

"Thank you for letting me read your chemotherapy book. I found it very helpful in many ways. Whilst it is primarily directed at those with breast cancer, it still had relevance for me."

࿓

"You keep the spontaneity of your patients' comments and this makes it ring true and also lends itself to easy access."

࿓

"It was a good idea to target particular drugs and their side effects, so, for me, the section on Paclitaxel had lots to tell me and it was reassuring that other people had the same things happening to them as I did."

࿓

"I took lots of notes from the chapter on how to alleviate effects (diet, drinks, exercise etc.) and your suggestions for further reading were good."

࿓

"It is a little mine of valuable information, advice and tips, which one doesn't necessarily get from anywhere else. I would think most patients undergoing chemotherapy would find it a practical and supportive guide and be glad of it."

❧

"I think the whole thing is really interesting and would have been great to have available at the time I was first diagnosed."

❧

"The author of this book has been a neighbour and tennis sparring partner prior to my diagnosis, and although I would have hoped never to meet her in her professional capacity, has now been a source of strength and encouragement to me through her wealth of knowledge gained through years working and treating those with cancer. Having access to this book whilst on my road through operations, chemotherapy and radiotherapy has been invaluable. I can only cope with one stage at a time in my head so at first I was not ready to take on board all the information that was provided. But as each step progressed, it is a great reference point and very reassuring to know that what you are feeling emotionally and experiencing physically are the same or similar to other people. Any little tip that helps cope with this difficult time can only be a positive thing and the way it is written in bite-size sections means that you can dip in and out of it at each relevant stage without feeling overwhelmed."

My top 6 tips for patients

These are based on my thoughts, experiences and are just suggestions.

1. Listen to the people that can help you i.e. healthcare workers and recognised breast cancer sites. Their experience and support is invaluable, and is there to be accessed. No question will be too trivial.

2. Allow yourself to feel all the different emotions that come with this diagnosis. So many patients have said that they feel they have to be strong for everyone else when actually they feel the opposite. You are the most important person in this scenario; you need to look after yourself and accept help as and when you need it .

3. Take someone with you to your appointments to begin with. It really helps to have another set of ears and the support of friend/family member.

4. Eat little and often!

5. Access the charities that can give you therapies that can make you feel better. For example, many patients have commented on how

much they've benefitted from reflexology, mindfulness counselling, the 'Look Good Feel Better' sessions with Macmillan Cancer. NB: whilst having chemotherapy, it's advisable to avoid acupuncture due to the risk of infection.

6. Give yourself time to recover after the treatment has finished. Over the years, I've seen many women rush the recovery process which has made it longer.

Glossary

Adjuvant therapy: Additional treatment given after initial treatment to remove or treat cancer in order to reduce the risk that cancer will come back in the future. Adjuvant therapy may include chemotherapy, radiation therapy, hormone therapy, targeted therapy or biological therapy.

Anti–emetics: Drugs which are used to prevent and/or treat nausea and vomiting.

Anti-nausea: See 'anti–emetics'.

Aromatherapy: A type of complementary medicine in which small amounts of oils extracted from plants are massaged into the skin.

Breast care nurse: A trained nurse who specialises in the care of patients with breast cancer and other breast conditions.

Cancer: A group of diseases characterised by the uncontrolled growth of abnormal cells which can invade healthy tissues in the body and spread to different parts of the body. There are more than 200 different types of cancer.

Chemotherapy (also known as cytotoxics): Drugs which are given to treat cancer by destroying cancer cells. Chemotherapy is most commonly given directly into the vein from a syringe or a drip but a few chemotherapy drugs are now available in tablet form.

Cold cap machine: Some chemotherapy drugs cause damage to hair follicles resulting in reversible hair loss. Using a cold cap (also known as scalp cooling) can reduce this hair loss. The cap is placed on the head and fitted closely before being switched on and then acts by reducing the temperature of the scalp a few degrees immediately before, during and after the administration of chemotherapy. This in turn reduces the blood flow to hair follicles which may prevent or minimise hair loss. For more information, see www.paxmanscalpcooling.com

Consultant: Doctors who have been qualified for a minimum of eight years and have completed all the training required to specialise in a specific field of hospital medicine or surgery.

Core needle biopsy: A procedure in which a needle is used to remove several cylinder-shaped samples of tissue from the area of the body under investigation in order to provide a diagnosis. For core biopsies of the breast, the needle is inserted about three to six times during an ultrasound examination so that the doctor can get enough samples. Usually this procedure does not leave a scar, but there can be a small amount of bruising after the procedure. You may also hear this test referred to as a 'needle biopsy' or 'tru-cut needle biopsy'.

Cystitis: Irritation of the bladder resulting in a frequent need to pass urine and/or stinging when passing urine. This is most commonly caused by an infection but rarely can be caused by irritation from a chemotherapy drug.

Diagnosis: The process of identifying the medical condition which is affecting a patient. As well as taking a full history of the symptoms, this may involve a doctor performing a physical examination and/or organising investigations.

Eczema: Inflammation of the skin resulting in redness and soreness with itching and sometimes scaling and blistering.

General Practitioner (GP): A doctor with a broad medical knowledge who works in a community surgery rather than a hospital and is responsible for referring a patient to hospital for specialist care when required.

GI symptoms: Symptoms related to the gastrointestinal system which includes the gullet (oesophagus), stomach and/or bowel.

Heartburn: A burning pain in the centre of the chest, which may travel from the tip of the breastbone to the throat and which is the result of irritation of the gullet or stomach. It may be triggered by eating rich or spicy food, drinking alcohol or by certain drugs.

Hickman or central line: A long thin tube which is inserted into the chest to provide a route by which to administer chemotherapy and take blood tests. The line is put in by a doctor or nurse under a local anaesthetic. Central lines are sometimes called skin-tunnelled central venous catheters, Hickman or Groshong lines. The central line can usually stay in until the full course of chemotherapy is completed.

Laxatives: Drugs used to treat constipation (difficulty in opening the bowels).

Lymph nodes: Structures found at intervals along the vessels which carry the lymph fluid around the body system. Their job is to filter out and trap bacteria, viruses, cancer cells, and other unwanted substances, and to make sure they are safely eliminated from the body. Lymph nodes can become enlarged when a patient has an infection and when they contain cancer cells.

Malignant: A medical term primarily used to refer to an abnormal growth or swelling (tumour) which is made up of cancer cells. Malignant or cancer cells are potentially able to spread from their original location to form secondary tumours in other parts of the body; these secondary tumours are known as metastases.

Mammogram: An investigation in which X-rays are used to produce images of the breast in order to detect abnormal growths or changes in the breast tissue.

Metastases: Tumours or cancer deposits which are caused by the spread of the primary cancer to other parts of the body. These are also known as secondary tumours or 'secondaries'. Metastases can occur in any part of the body but most frequently occur in the bones, lungs, liver, skin and brain, and are usually multiple.

Mucositis: Inflammation or irritation of any of the soft tissues lining the mouth, gullet, stomach, or bowel resulting in soreness and temporary damage to the tissues. This can occur as a side effect of chemotherapy and some radiotherapy treatments.

Nausea: The sensation of feeling sick.

Neutropenic: Low numbers of a certain type of white blood cells (neutrophils) circulating in the bloodstream resulting in a patient being at a higher risk of catching an infection.

Oncologist: A doctor who specialises in treating cancer. Medical oncologists specialise in using anti-cancer drugs whilst clinical oncologists specialise in using radiotherapy treatments.

Oral thrush: A fungal infection of the mouth which causes white furring of the tongue and an unpleasant taste. This is a common side effect of chemotherapy treatments and is readily treated with medications.

Portacath: A type of central line in which one end of a long hollow tube (usually made of silicon rubber) is placed into one of the large veins in the body, which is attached to a round, hollow port positioned beneath the skin on the front of the chest, just below collar bone. You will be able to feel the port as a lump under your skin. A special needle is used to access the port in order to take blood tests and administer injections including chemotherapy drugs, which can be given via the port.

Prognosis: An assessment of the likely outcome of a disease which may include an approximate estimate of life expectancy.

Radiotherapy: The use of high dose X-rays to destroy cancer cells within the area of the body that the X-ray beam is aimed at. Radiotherapy is usually administered as a course of repeated short treatments.

Reiki healing: A form of complementary therapy that uses touch and/or visualisation techniques with the aim of improving the flow of energy in an individual.

Sentinel node biopsy: A process in which the first main lymph node to drain a specific area of the body (e.g. breast) is identified by special imaging techniques. The surgeons then remove this lymph node and check it for cancer cells to determine whether more extensive removal of the lymph nodes in the area is required.

Steroids (also called corticosteroids): Substances that are naturally produced in the body which help reduce inflammation and control different functions in our bodies, such as the immune system or the way the body uses food. Steroids can also be man-made and given as drugs as part of your cancer treatment. Steroids can be taken as tablets or liquids by mouth or by injection and help to prevent sickness and to reduce the risk of allergic reactions.

Surgeon: A doctor who specialises in treating illnesses or injuries by physically removing or repairing tissues in an operation.

Tumeric: A yellow powder derived from the ginger plant family which is primarily used for flavouring and colouring in Asian cookery.

Common supportive drugs (this list is by no means exhaustive)

Aprepitant: used to treat or prevent sickness or vomiting

Codeine: used to treat pain and to slow down diarrhoea

Cyclizine: used to treat or prevent sickness or vomiting

Dexamethasone: a steroid used to prevent sickness and vomiting, prevent allergic reactions and reduce inflammation

Domperidone: used to treat or prevent sickness or vomiting

Loperamide: used to treat diarrhoea

Magnesium hydroxide: used to treat constipation

Metoclopramide: used to treat or prevent sickness or vomiting

Movicol: used to treat constipation

Nystatin: used to treat thrush in the mouth

Ondansetron: used to treat or prevent sickness or vomiting

Paracetamol: A drug used to treat pain and fever

Pyridoxine (vitamin B6): used to treat soreness of the hands and feet caused by some chemotherapy drugs

Sucralfate: used to help sore mouths or mouth ulcers

References

Cancer Research UK
www.cancerresearchuk.org

Chemotherapy
For information on chemotherapy, see
www.macmillan.org.uk

AC refers to Adriamyacin or Doxorubicin and
Cyclophosphamide

EC refers to Epirubicin Cyclophosphamide

FEC chemotherapy refers to Fluorouracil
see Epirubicin Cyclophosphamide

T refers to Taxotere or Docetaxel

Taxane Paclitaxel   see www.macmillan.org.uk

Radiotherapy   see www.macmillan.org.uk

Hormonal treatment

Tamoxifen   see www.macmillan.org.uk
Menopace   see www.vitabiotics.com/menopace

Monoclonal antibody treatment
Herceptin   see www.macmillan.org.uk

Central lines/Implantable ports
Hickman   see www.macmillan.org.uk

"Central lines are long, hollow tubes made from silicone rubber. They are also called skin-tunnelled central venous catheters. Some catheters that are used are Hickman ® or Groshong ®. Hickman and Groshong are registered trademarks of CR Bard Inc, or an affiliate.

"The central line is put in (tunnelled) under the skin of your chest and into a vein close by. One end of the line goes into a large vein just above your heart. The other end comes out of your chest.

"The line is usually sealed with a special cap or bung. This can be attached to a drip or syringe containing your medication. There may be a clamp to keep the line closed when it's not being used.

"Sometimes it divides into two or three lines. This allows you to have different treatments at the same time."

Portacath   see www.macmillan.org.uk

"An implantable port is a thin, soft, hollow tube made of plastic. It's put into a vein in your chest or arm.

"It has an opening just under the skin. This is called the port. The port is a disc about 2.5-4cm (1-1.5in) in diameter. It can be used to give medicine into your vein, or to take blood.

"The tube is usually put in (tunnelled) under the skin of your chest or sometimes in your arm. One end of the tube goes into a large vein just above your heart. The other end connects with the port. This goes under the skin on your upper chest or arm. You'll be able to see and feel a small bump underneath your skin."

Nausea and vomiting

Good n Natural Ginger Root Capsules 550mg   www.hollandandbarrett.com

Preserved Ginger   www.realfoods.co.uk/product/2583/organic-fresh-ginger

Dorset Ginger   www.dorsetginger.com

Jacob's Cream Crackers

Constipation

Magnesium Hydroxide   www.chemistdirect.co.uk/magnesium-hydroxide-mixture/prd-ba

Movicol   www.chemistdirect.co.uk/brands/movicol/bnd-2n7

Senna   www.lloydspharmacy.com/en/lloyds pharmacy-senna-tablets-60-tablets

Taste changes/Sore mouth

Aloe vera toothpaste   www.hollandandbarrett.com

Bonjela   www.bonjela.co.uk

Chlorexidine Gluconate Antiseptic Mouthwash www.superdrug.com/Superdrug/Superdrug-Chlorhexidine-Mouthwash-300ml/p/232054

Corsadyl Mouthwash   www.corsodyl.co.uk

Oralden   www.waitrose.com/shop/ProductView-10317-10001-31511-Oraldene+mouthwash

Rinstead have been discontinued and an alternative pastille is Iglu Sugar Free Pastille. See www.boots.com

Manuka Honey 25 +   www.amazon.co.uk

Hair loss/Scalp care

Annabandana   www.annabandana.co.uk

Accessorize   http://uk.accessorize.com/

Buff snoods   www.amazon.co.uk

Baker Boy Hats   www.bakerboy-hats.stylight.co.uk

Rosemary and Cedarwood Neals Yard Hair Treatment   www.nealsyardremedies.com

Skin problems

The Body Shop   www.thebodyshop.co.uk

E45 Cream   www.superdrug.com

Epaderm   www.amazon.co.uk

Liquid Piriton   www.lloydspharmacy.com/en/piriton-syrup-150ml

Palmers Oil   www.boots.com

Vaseline

Dr Organics   www.hollandandbarrett.com

Eucerin www.boots.com

Udderly Smooth Foot Cream www.wiggle.co.uk

Miscellaneous

Neutropenic see www.macmillan.org.uk

Cystitis http://www.nhs.uk/conditions/cystitis/ Pages/Introduction.aspx

Walk & Talk Refer to local support websites

Look Good Feel Better workshops at local Macmillan Centres and hospitals. To find your local workshop, visit www.lookgoodfeelbetter.co.uk

Macmillan Centres to find your local centre, visit www.macmillan.org.uk

Wessex Cancer Trust see www.wessexcancer.org.uk

Bristol Cancer Centre/Penny Brohn Centre see www.pennybrohn.org.uk

Amoena underwear see www.amoena.com

Throat Coat Tea   see www.revital.co.uk

LifeMel Honey   see http://www.nirvanahealthfood.com/life-mel-honey-113gms.html

Spatone Iron supplement   see www.boots.com

Aloe vera juice shot

Books

Breast Reconstruction: Your Choice (Class Health) by Dick Rainsbury and Ginny Straker (Class Publishing, 2008)

Healthy Eating During Chemotherapy (Healthy Eating Series) by Jose van Mil (Kyle Cathie, 2008)

The Juice Master – Keeping it Simple by Jason Vale (Harper Thorsons, 2007). www.juicemaster.com

Your Brain After Chemo: A Practical Guide to Lifting the Fog and Getting Back Your Focus byDan Silverman and Idelle Davidson (Da Capo Lifelong Books, 2010)

Your Life In Your Hands: Understand, Prevent and Overcome Breast Cancer and Ovarian Cancer by Professor Jane Plant (Virgin Books, 2007)

Complementary medicines

See http://www.cancerresearchuk.org/about-cancer/
cancers-in-general/treatment/complementary-
alternative/

Breast cancer charities

Breast Cancer Care   www.breastcancercare.org.uk

Breast Cancer Haven   www.breastcancerhaven.org.uk

The Lavender Trust at Breast Cancer Care. Raises
money specifically to fund information and support
for younger women with breast cancer.
www.lavendertrust.org.uk

Macmillan Cancer Support   www.macmillan.org.uk

Lightning Source UK Ltd.
Milton Keynes UK
UKOW06f1416041216
289178UK00001B/5/P